the 5 MINUTE FACE

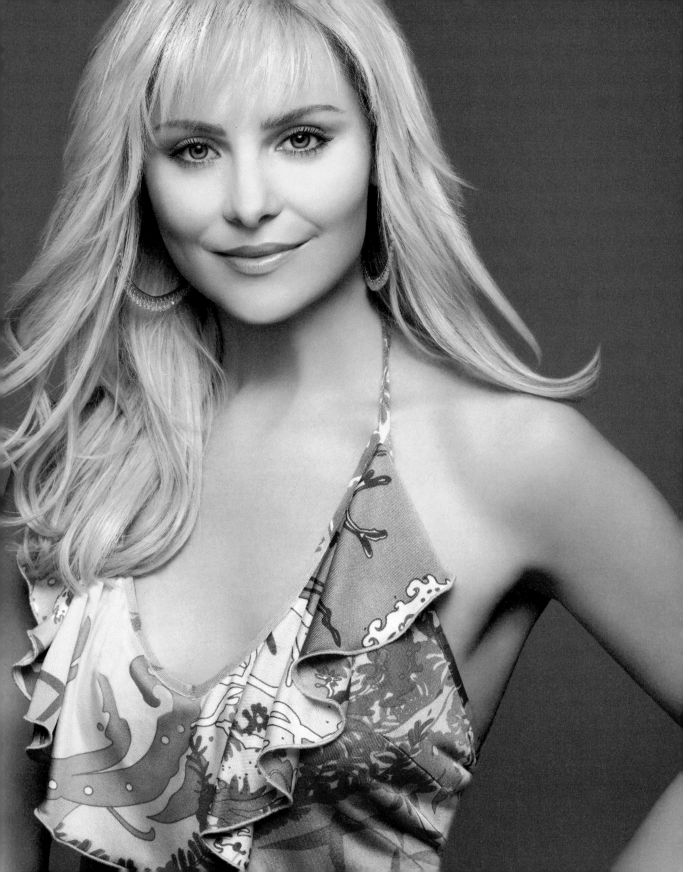

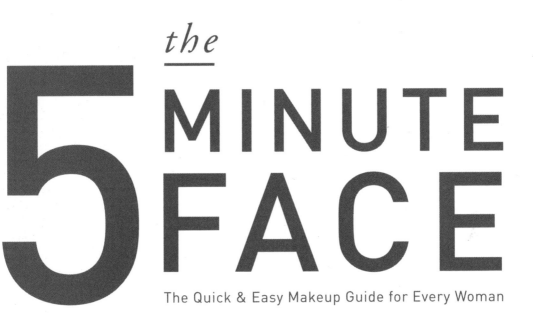

the 5 MINUTE FACE

The Quick & Easy Makeup Guide for Every Woman

CARMINDY

BEAUTY PHOTOGRAPHY BY PALMA KOLANSKY

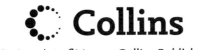

Collins

An Imprint of HarperCollinsPublishers

All model and author photography by Palma Kolansky; all photography of makeup swatches by Devon Jarvis.

HarperCollins books may be purchased for educational, business, or sales promotional use. For information please write: Special Markets Department, HarperCollins Publishers, 10 East 53rd Street, New York, NY 10022.

Designed by Kris Tobiassen

Library of Congress Cataloging-in-Publication Data

Carmindy.
   The 5-minute face : the quick and easy makeup guide for every woman / Carmindy.—1st ed.
     p.   cm.
   ISBN 13: 978-0-06-123826-0
   ISBN 10:0-06-123826-0
   1. Beauty, Personal. 2. Face—Care and hygiene. 3. Skin—Care and hygiene. 4. Cosmetics. I. Title.

RA778.C2167 2007
646.7'2—dc22

                        2006049701

08 09 10 11 */RRD 10 9 8 7 6

To my beautiful mother, Julie, my inspiration,
and my father, Jack, who always encouraged me
to follow my passions in life and create my
own destiny. I love you!

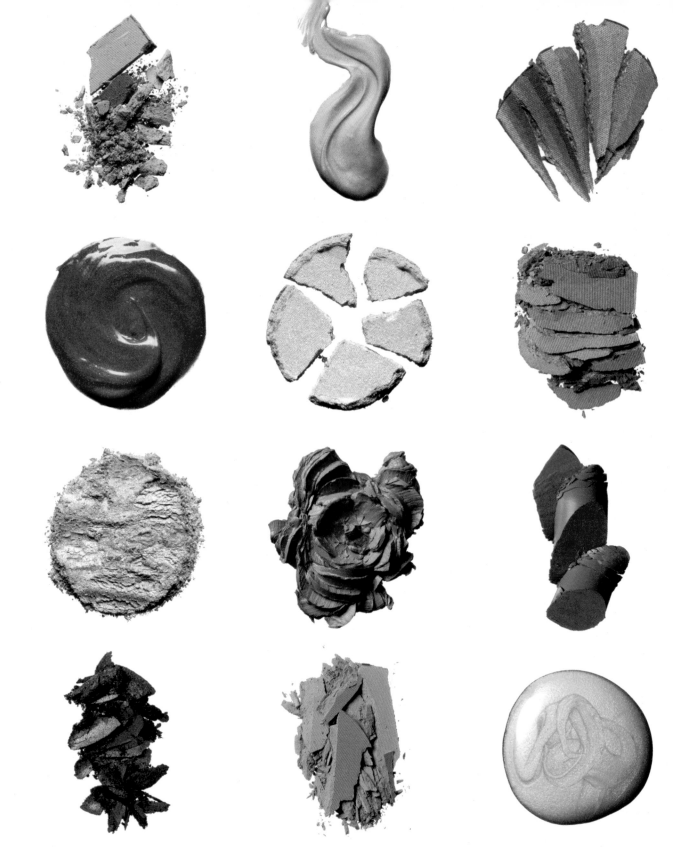

CONTENTS

the 5 MINUTE FACE

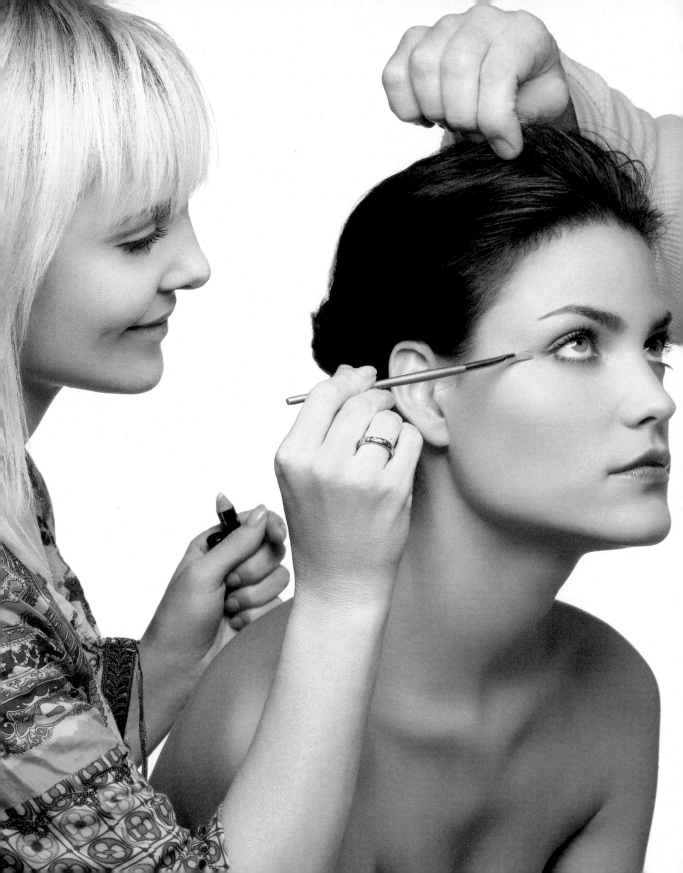

NOT SURE WHAT MAKEUP TO WEAR?

No wonder. I've noticed a bizarre trend in recent years. The more we have advanced as women, the more insecure we have become. When it comes to our looks, we only see what's wrong with us, how we can fix it, and how we can achieve someone else's idea of perfection. And we are deluged by that promise to make lashes longer, to eliminate cellulite, and to erase wrinkles!

I believe we must retrain our brains. Instead of searching for what is wrong, we need to focus on what's right—what we *already* possess that is beautiful. Women constantly ask me questions like, "Carmindy, how do I make my lips look larger?" Meanwhile the woman asking has the *most extraordinary* brown eyes I have ever seen. She doesn't even realize this because she's obsessed with making her lips look huge. What a shame!

Here's my philosophy: When it comes to using makeup, I believe in using the right products in the right places to highlight your best features, instead of piling on products to re-create your face or hide perceived flaws. I don't believe that women are flawed or that there is any set standard of beauty they MUST meet. In my fifteen years in the beauty business as a makeup artist for countless magazine and advertising shoots, and now as the makeup host on The Learning Channel's *What Not to Wear* television show, I've worked with models, celebrities, stay-at-home moms—women from all walks of life. There is beauty in everyone, and I help each person see it.

How? For one thing, I show them how simple makeup application can be. I apply it like a watercolor painting: I use sheer washes of color that allow one's natural beauty to shine through. Relearning how to use makeup to enhance your features will help you embrace and celebrate your glowing skin, lovely lips, sparkling eyes—whatever you possess that is truly beautiful. Your insecurities will vanish, and using makeup will be a lot more fun.

That's why I've written this book, *The 5-Minute Face,* and why I've spent so much time on this approach—I want makeup to be a fast and foolproof way for all women to maximize their beauty potential. And I want all those women out there to see beauty in themselves and to celebrate the way they look. It's amazing how one seemingly simple tip can unleash a whole wave of self-esteem. Now it's time to embrace your natural beauty, enhance your best features, and enlighten your sense of self.

I BECAME INTERESTED IN MAKEUP WHEN I WAS FIFTEEN YEARS OLD. MY mother was a watercolor artist, and I would sit with her and watch her paint for hours. It was also about that time that I remember digging up old photos of my grandmother and my mother from their modeling days. I became fascinated with those glamorous images. Seeing my interest, my mother bought me a subscription to *Elle* magazine and I was *hooked*! I wanted to look like the women on those pages, and I wanted to make everyone else look that way, too: clean, healthy, gorgeous.

For Christmas one year, I asked my father to build me a Hollywood-style makeup mirror—the ones with the big lightbulbs all around—and a director's chair. I began doing makeup for friends and neighbors, re-creating what I saw on those fashion pages and incorporating some of the techniques I had learned watching my mother paint.

That became one of my hallmarks: my "watercolor" approach to makeup. The more I followed this method, the more I realized how gorgeous skin looks with minimal makeup. I also mastered the art of choosing just one great feature to showcase. For me, it's about finding the positive and playing it up. And I'm going to share all of my techniques with you.

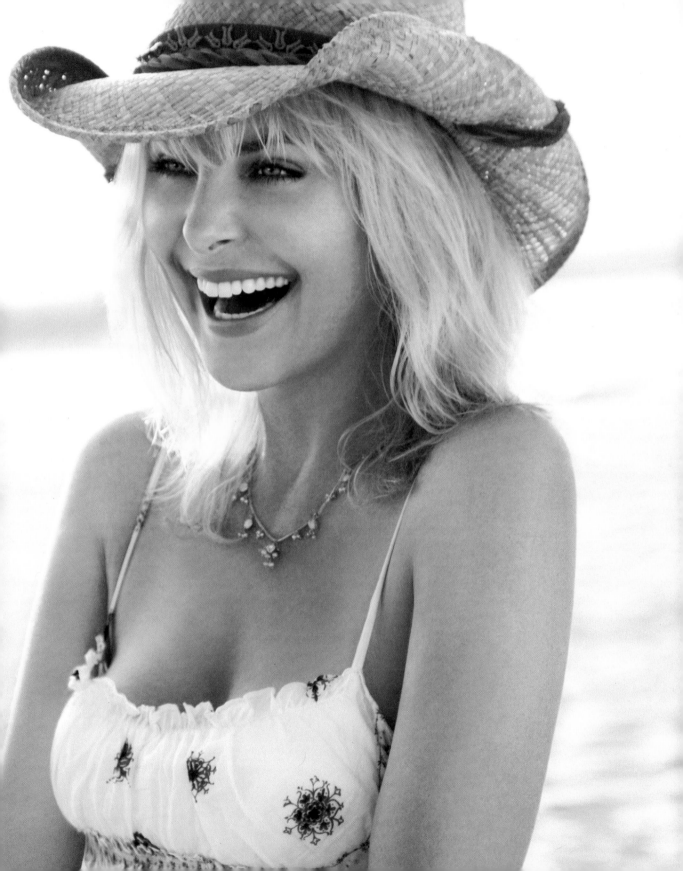

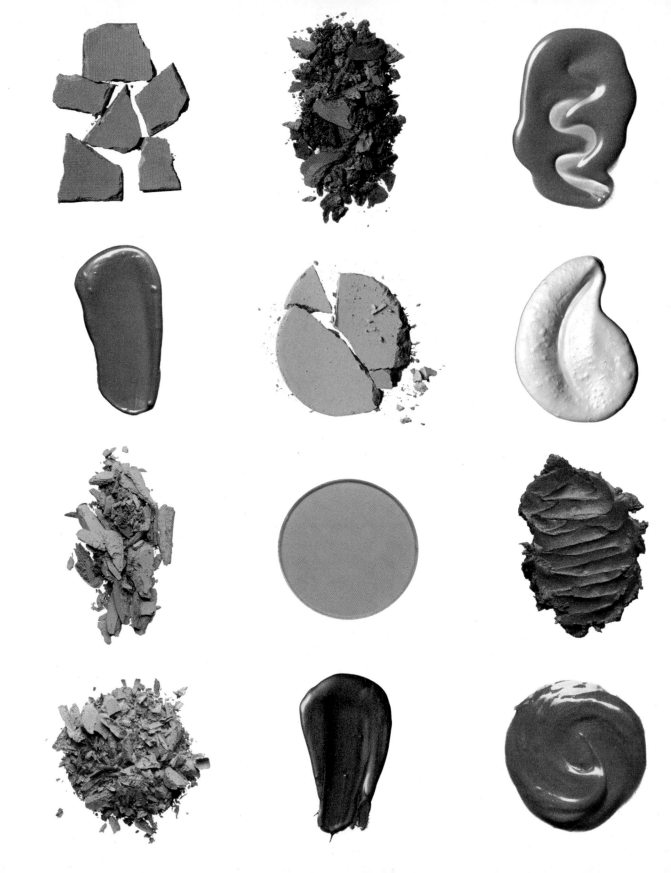

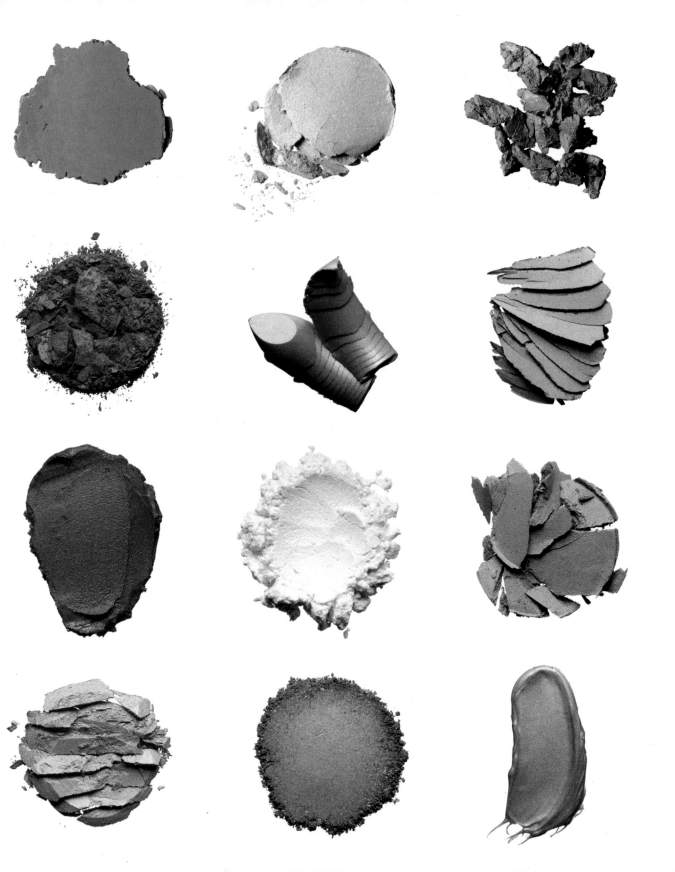

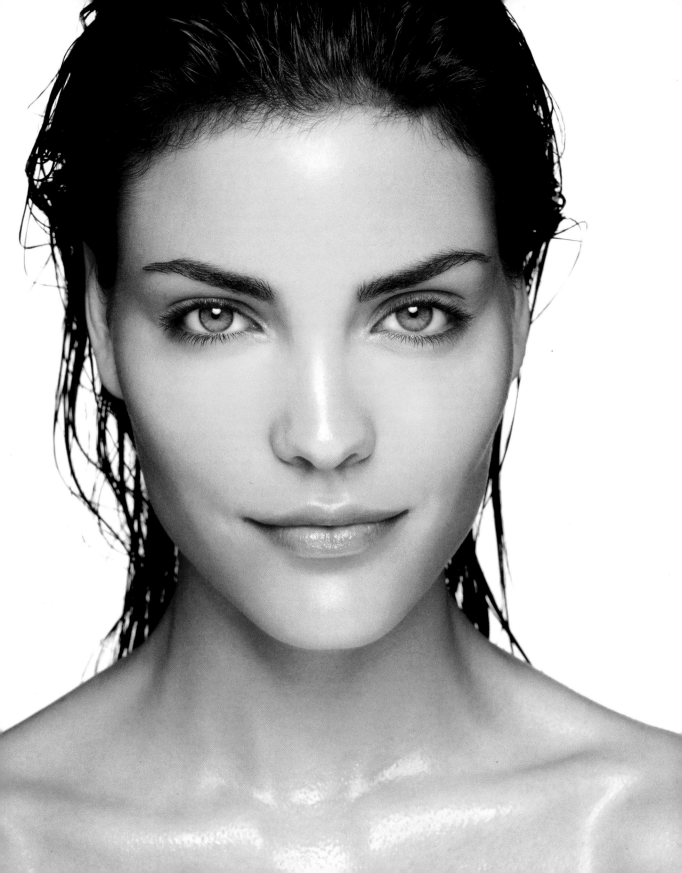

chapter one

SKIN ESSENTIALS

One of my main goals when I apply makeup is to let my clients' skin show through; I don't cake on foundation or concealer. But in order for skin to be in its best possible shape, you've got to treat it well. It isn't hard. Just find the right cleanser, wash your skin in the morning and before bed, and use moisturizer regularly (a daytime lotion with SPF and something richer, like a cream or serum, at night) to make your complexion radiant. And when skin glows, so will the rest of you. Below, find your skin type and take note of the easy-care steps.

OILY SKIN

Oily skin tends to break out more, even into your forties, but regular cleansing can go a long way to keep your face clear. By about age thirty-five, you may notice that oil output slows and skin is more normal. And, good news: that extra oil keeps your skin looking soft and youthful longer than other skin types.

- **THE RIGHT CLEANSER** For *day*, use a *foaming gel cleanser*. The lather will help break down sebum (skin's natural oil), and since foamers typically don't leave extra moisturizers behind the way creamy cleansers do, they are your best bet for *keeping skin clear*.

■ **THE RIGHT MOISTURIZER** Use an *oil-free lotion*. A lot of women assume that if their skin is oily, they should skip moisturizer. Not true. Your skin will feel dehy-drated and will overcompensate by producing more oil. Trick it into thinking it has enough moisture by using an oil-free formula. This will also function like a primer to even skin texture so foundation goes on smoothly, which will help makeup last longer. *At night,* apply an oil-free lotion with *alpha hydroxy acids* to exfoliate skin and keep pores clear. Use this regularly and you'll notice softer, smoother skin and fewer breakouts.

NORMAL SKIN–COMBINATION SKIN

The truth? **Normal skin *is* combination skin!** Yup—we all have more oil glands along our T-zone (the forehead, nose, and chin) than on the rest of our face, and every one of us sees shine there. Normal skin has a dewier T-zone midday, but few pimples. It can teeter toward oily or dry.

■ **THE RIGHT CLEANSER** Use a *daily liquid cleanser*. Liquid cleansers tend to be mild and well balanced, so they will wash away dirt and oil but won't overdry your skin.

■ **THE RIGHT MOISTURIZER** Use *lightweight lotions*. Lotions will give you the perfect amount of moisture without being too heavy. *At night*, use the lightweight lotion and add a cream formula on your drier areas. This is the ideal time to apply a rich cream that may be too greasy for daytime use—your skin will be glowing when you wake up!

DRY SKIN

Dry skin has its pros and cons. Pores are usually less visible and you rarely get a blemish, but if you skimp on moisturizer, lines can stand out more and skin can look flat.

- THE RIGHT CLEANSER Choose a *creamy cleanser*. This type of product will offer lightweight hydration. Keep in mind that dry skin needs moisture added to every beauty step, including cleansers and foundations.

- THE RIGHT MOISTURIZER Use a cream that will replace lost moisture to keep your skin soft and supple. Try to remember this five-minute rule: if skin feels tight five minutes after applying moisturizer, your formula isn't rich enough. Try applying the cream to damp skin in order to lock in water for maximum softness. *At night*, add a super-rich cream with antioxidant vitamins. Just keeping your skin well hydrated will plump it up for a youthful, fresh look. Tip: Use a humidifier in the winter. You'll be amazed at what it will do for your skin (and hair, which may also be dry). Tap on a rich eye cream and lip balm at night, as well.

SENSITIVE SKIN QUICK TIPS

No matter why you have sensitive skin, these steps should help you manage it:

- Avoid fragranced skin care products or makeup.

- Wash your skin with cool water. Cold or hot water can irritate delicate complexions.

- Say no to scrubs. They can be too harsh.

- Always spot test. Using skin by your jaw or inner elbow, test a product for a day or two to see if it bothers your complexion.

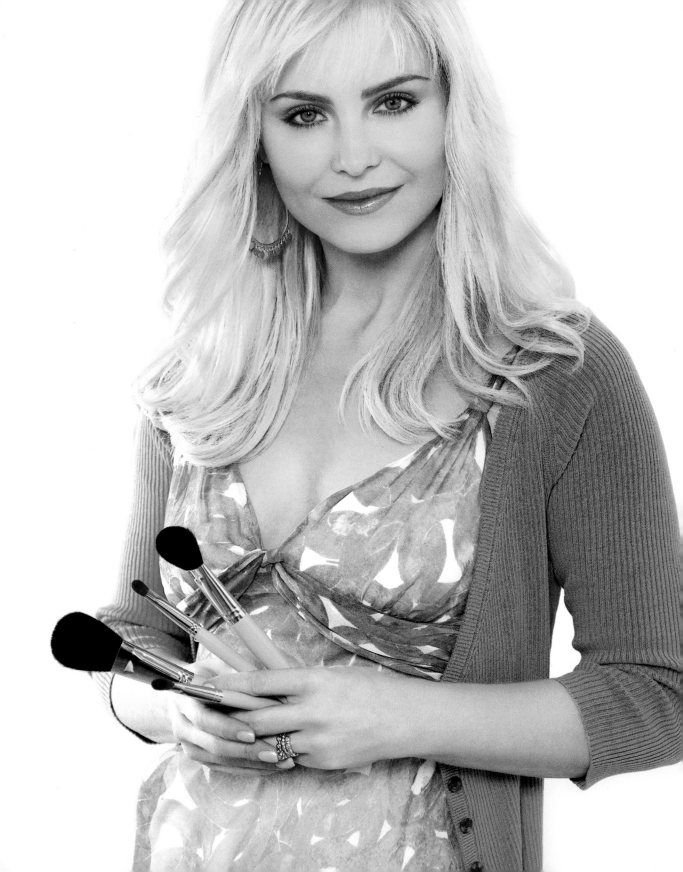

THE EASIEST, BEST WAY TO REMOVE MASCARA

For convenience, nothing beats premoistened makeup remover cloths or pads. The difference between these and ones labeled "face cleansing cloths" are that makeup remover cloths have oilier ingredients that better break down mascara's waxes (including waterproof brands) with no scrubbing required. Tip: remove mascara gently by closing your upper lids and swiping the cloth or pad in a smooth, light, downward stroke—grinding it in can cause lashes to fall out.

Eye Cream: Worth the Splurge

Sure, you can apply face lotion under your eyes. But dedicated eye creams are made to be gentler, with nonirritating ingredients that won't sting this sensitive area or cause tears. I'm not one for extra stuff rattling around my makeup case, but this splurge is worth it. If you have puffiness, look for formulas that firm. Circles? Try products with vitamin K.

Toner Talk

Twenty years ago, toners were made of witch hazel, alcohol, or both. They were marketed to banish excess oil, and they did—too well! Most of us who used them were left with parched skin. Not surprisingly, they fell out of favor and were viewed as an unnecessary step. Today, gentler versions are available. Botanical toners are refreshing and smell especially good. Myself, I love simple rose water (it's hydrating and calming) or cucumber water (it's a mild astringent and good for oily skin). Both can be found at health food stores. Tip: pour rose or cucumber water into a spray bottle, store in your fridge, and spritz away to rejuvenate skin on a hot day.

Sunscreen Smarts

I am diligent about wearing sunscreen, and you should be, too. It is the single best way to keep skin looking young and healthy. Not convinced? Here's what regular use will help prevent: fine lines, deep wrinkles, discoloration (like light or dark patches), roughness, crepey texture, sagginess, broken capillaries, and of course, skin cancer. That's quite a list! I use SPF

15 for intermittent exposure—when I'm running errands from store to store—and SPF 30 or 45 at the beach or when I'm out for a bike ride or hike. Read labels and choose a formula that's "broad spectrum." It will protect you against both ultraviolet A (UVA) and B (UVB) rays. Choosing daytime moisturizers with built-in suncreens will also save you time in the morning, cutting out an extra step.

EXFOLIATORS

Exfoliators remove dead cells, as well as grime and oil that collect on the skin's surface and in pores. Get rid of that useless muck and your face will look soft and glowing. But use too many types of exfoliators at once or too often, and your skin will appear dry and flaky instead of radiant and soft. You can't go wrong with a gentle AHA product. Glycolic, malic, and lactic acids are common AHAs, and you'll find them in daytime and nighttime moisturizers, foundations, washes, and more. Choose one AHA product and you'll be set. If you are in your mid-thirties or beyond, consider a **glycolic peel,** which has the effect of two weeks' worth of daily glycolic cream in one shot. Glycolic peels smooth skin's surface, minimize lines, and fade brown sunspots. They're meant to be done in a series of six to twelve treatments, a little at a time. (Immediately after applying, your skin may look pink, like you've just worked out.) I get a series of treatments every year to perk up my skin; it glows afterward like you won't believe. A dermatologist's office is the best place to receive a glycolic peel, because a doctor can use a stronger formula than what you'll get from a day spa or home kit. Remember, to keep lasting results, use sunscreen every day.

DON'T FORGET YOUR LIPS!

Lips need TLC, too. To make them kissably smooth, apply a plain, creamy lip balm before bed every night. It will add back softness you lose during the day. To smooth chapping, rub on balm before you hop in the shower. Immediately after, gently buff lips with a few pinches of sugar and a wet terry washcloth. Easy!

BEAUTIFY YOUR BODY!

Want fabulously sexy skin all over your body? Who doesn't! These easy tricks will leave you touchably soft and radiant from your neck to your toes.

My Instant (and Cheap!) Body-Glow Secret

I love to customize my own body lotion. I spend far less than I would for a fancy lotion, and I get exactly what I want. Here's my secret: I buy a big jug of inexpensive, unscented lotion from the drugstore, then add drops of my favorite essential oil (like coconut or jasmine, which you can find at health food stores). Next I add a squeeze of liquid or cream shimmer (a luminizer that most cosmetics companies offer). Then shake it all up, and wow! I not only smell yummy, but my body is soft and luminous. What's more, the glow from the shimmer (aim for a subtle gleam, not an obvious glittery look) makes your muscle tone stand out, even if you don't have much. Who doesn't want that? Ever since I started to wear my own lotion, I've received all sorts of compliments about my skin. You will too. Tip: store lotion near your bathtub or shower stall—it's the only way to guarantee you'll use it regularly.

Self-tanners

In addition to using my shimmery lotion religiously, I love a self-tanner. Sometimes I use it year-round, applying a lighter shade in the cooler months and a darker one in summer. I'm fair, so I never go darker than a medium shade; a deep tropical bronze would look too fake on me. A rule of thumb for all skin colors: choose brands that offer a few shade choices, and pick *one shade lighter* than you think you need. Trust me, it's the right one.

HOW TO APPLY YOUR "TAN" LIKE A PRO

- Exfoliate skin in the shower with a body scrub, loofah, or scrubby gloves, and shave your legs. The smoother skin is, the better the "tan" will look.

- Don't apply moisturizer to skin. It can prevent the self-tanning formula from taking hold and can result in spottiness.

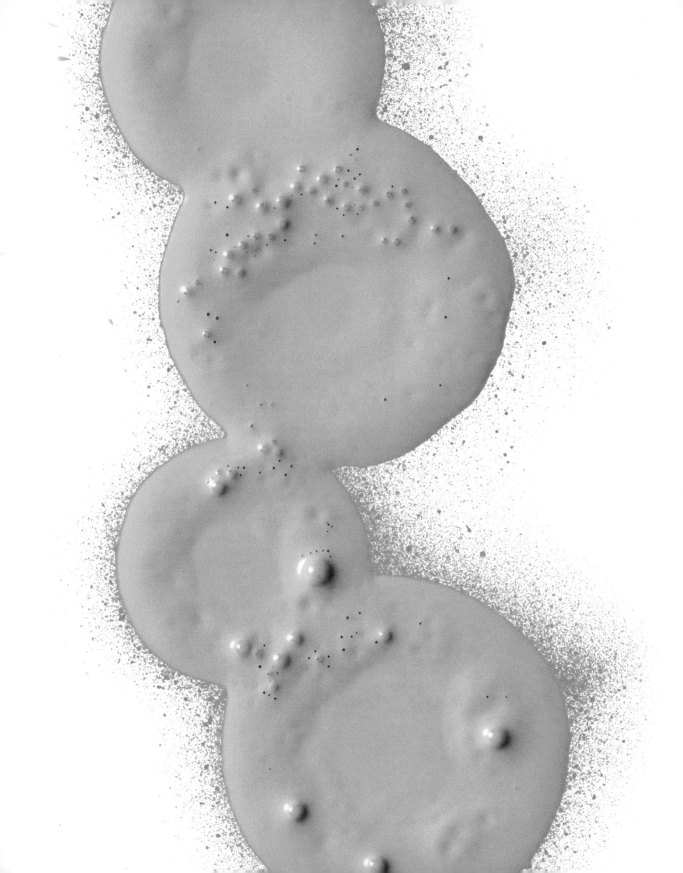

- When skin is 100 percent dry, apply your self-tanner evenly. Work in every zone to ensure you cover all areas.

- Move from head to toes and apply with fingers tightly closed (spreading self-tanner with splayed fingers can leave you with streaks).

- Use light, circular strokes for evenness.

- Don't tan the sides or heels of your feet—the thick skin there will soak up the formula. Instead, make your "tan" fade gradually from your shins to your feet, by blending down softly.

- After applying, immediately scrub your hands with soap, water, and sugar so your palms don't turn dark. Don't forget to scrub between your fingers and your cuticles!

- Last, take a barely-damp washcloth and buff your knees, elbows, around your jaw line, ankles, feet, and wrists to blend and soften the color there and to avoid demarcation lines. If you feel the need to go darker, repeat the process the next day, and so on, until you get the desired color.

Fast Fix

In the shower, buff skin with a handful of regular white sugar—it's an inexpensive and amazing face and body scrub. To help erase self-tanning streaks, add a teaspoon of lemon juice.

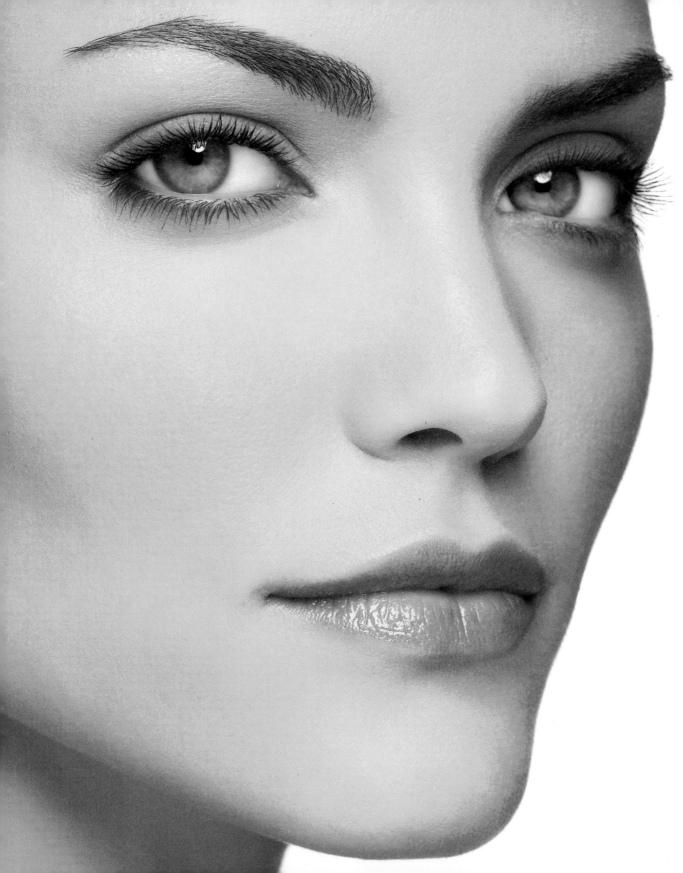

chapter two

GET BROWS THAT WOW

Any makeup artist will tell you that the brows frame the face. When they are groomed properly, your eyes will stand out more and your whole face will look more balanced. A perfect arch allows you to leave the house feeling a lot more comfortable wearing less makeup. *Never* shape your brow based on a photo of someone else's eyebrow shape. You have your own unique brow shape, and your look needs to be specially tailored to your face. As a general rule, thicker brows work best if you have a prominent bone structure; go with thinner brows on a small-featured face.

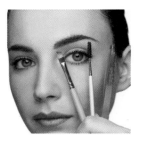

TOOLBOX: To create the perfect brow, you'll need a pair of quality tweezers, manicure scissors, and a brow brush; a brow pencil, powder, or brow groomer; a mirror, good light, and plenty of time. Don't rush!

FOUR STEPS TO PERFECT BROWS, EVERY TIME

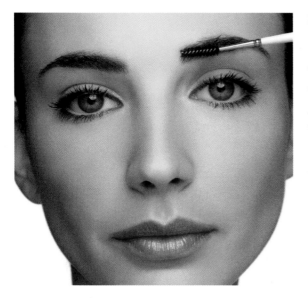

STEP 1: TRIM ANY WILD HAIRS.
Brush brows straight up. With manicure scissors (curved or straight—what matters are the tiny, snippy tips), trim any extra-long brow hairs that poke out of line. Note: if you're Asian, your brows may naturally fall downward. If that's the case, brush brows down and trim any hairs that fall below the natural shape, then brush them back up into place.

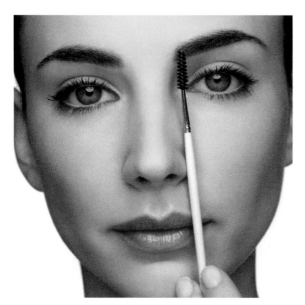

STEP 2: FIND YOUR STARTING POINT.
Rest a brow brush along the edge of your nose horizontally. One end should touch a nostril and the other should pass right over your forehead. Where the brow brush crosses your brow is where your brow line should start. Map out your other brow the same way, and pluck strays in the unibrow section that falls between these starting points.

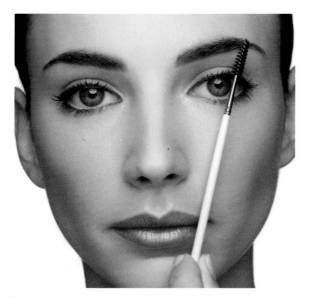

STEP 3: MAP OUT YOUR ARCH.

Starting by the edge of your lips, angle the brow brush diagonally so it passes right over the outer edge of your iris, the colored part of your eye. Where the brush crosses the brow is where your arch should be. Some women have a pointed arch; others have arches that are just slightly curved. Pluck any strays under this area so your natural arch is defined.

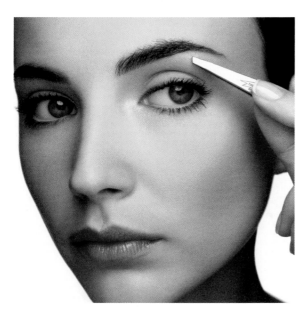

STEP 4: FIND YOUR ENDPOINT.

Again, shift your brow brush so it lays against your nostril and angle it back to the outer corner of your eye. This is where the endpoint of your brow should be. Nix strays that fall outside or below this area for a clean taper from arch to end. In general, full, long brows look more youthful and are easier to carry off than skinny brows.

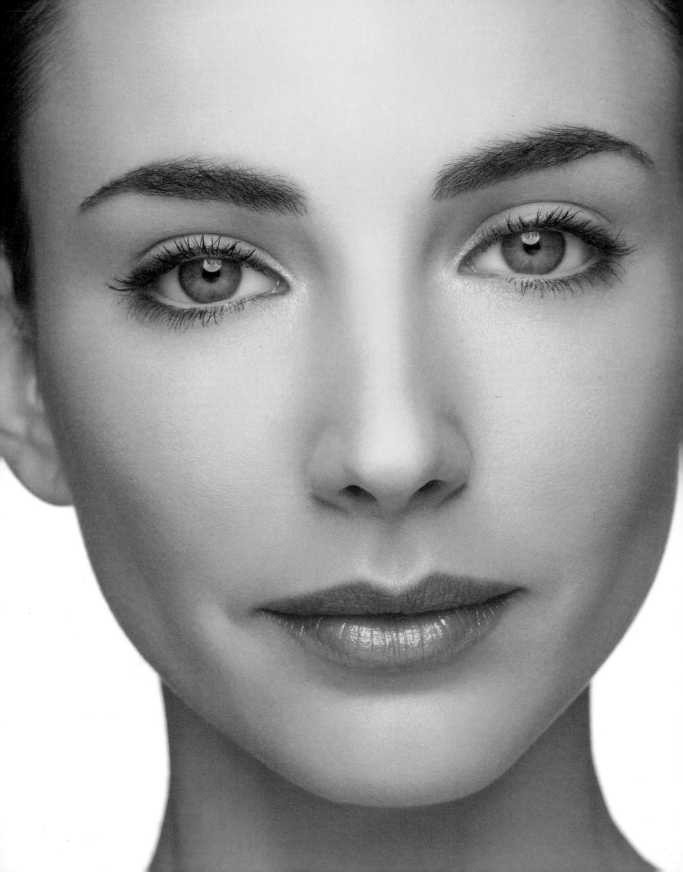

Bushy Beginners

If you have never plucked before and have a lot of stray hairs, outline your ideal, finished shape right over your existing brows using a white eyeliner pencil. Only pluck the hairs that fall outside of the white line, making your outline mistake proof. Just wipe off the white line when you're done, and your brows will be perfect.

Overpluckers Anonymous

Some of you get a little crazy when plucking your eyebrows and don't know when to stop. Careful ladies—brows may not grow back, and you could be condemning yourself to a lifetime of filling them back in. If you think you have compulsive tendencies, go ahead and splurge on a professional brow job (like waxing, tweezing, or threading) at a local salon.

Fast Fix

For models and celebrities, dying brows is normal. They do it to make their colored hair more believable but also to make their eyes pop. *Blondes* with light brows tend to go a shade darker (for eye definition) and *brunettes* usually go a shade lighter to soften their look. A professional colorist will usually do this for no charge while you're getting your roots touched up.

MYTH BUSTER #1

"Never pluck above the brow."

Not in my opinion. Some women are quite hairy above the brow. If you see excess hairs above your natural upper brow line, tweeze them!

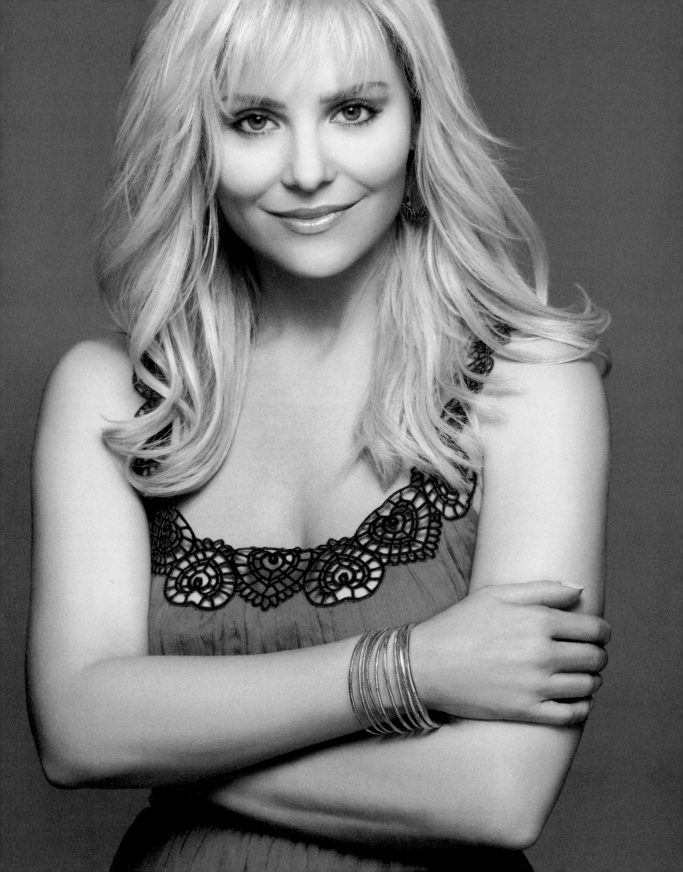

"If I pluck my brows they will grow back thicker."

Wrong! Hair follicles do not multiply. But if you pluck brow hairs straight out or in the opposite direction that they grow in naturally, they may start to grow in the wrong direction. This gives the illusion that they are thicker because they look wild.

Fast Fix

To minimize pain when tweezing, pluck right after showering, when your hair follicles are more open. Your hair will slide out more easily.

Finishing Touches: Brow Pencil, Powder, Groomer

No matter which brow finisher you choose, follow these color guidelines: *Redheads* should choose a light sable, which will add a little red color into normally pale brows. *Blondes* should choose the same shade as the darkest color in their hair (usually taupe). *Brunettes* and gals with *black hair* should choose one shade lighter than their natural hair color.

- **PENCIL** is easiest for novices because it offers control. Use it to fill in bald spots or to extend the brow slightly (brows can thin at the ends with age or from over-plucking). Make sure the pencil is sharp every time and use tiny hairlike strokes.

- **BROW POWDER** looks like eye shadow, but has a chalkier texture allowing it to stay put. Apply with a short, firm angled brush (often included with the powder) and again, use tiny hairlike strokes. Powder is the most natural looking brow finisher because it looks softer than pencil.

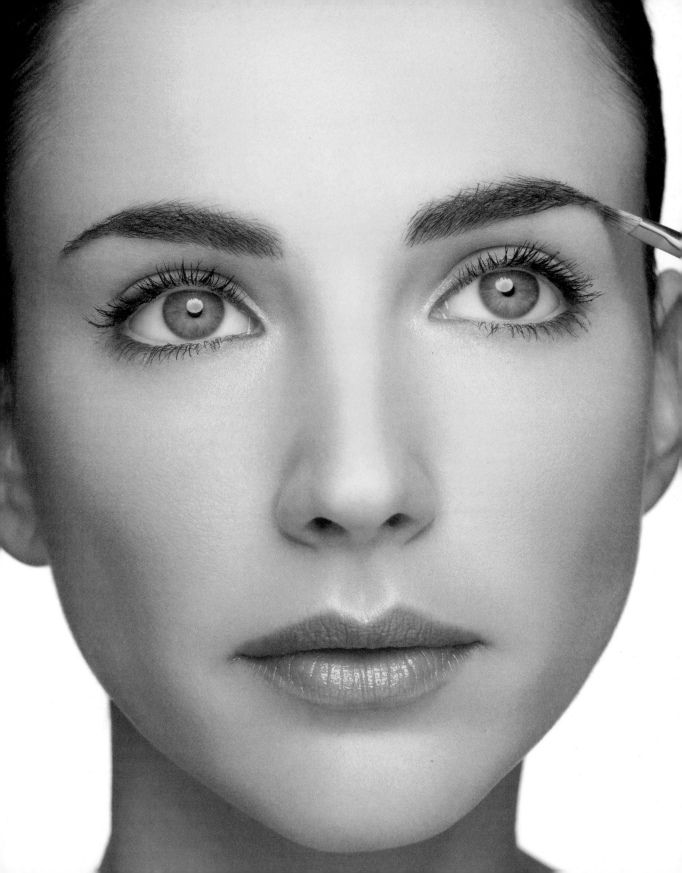

- **BROW GROOMER** looks like mascara, and can be clear or tinted. Brow groomers won't feel as stiff as mascara and will help keep your brow hairs in line if they tend to point down. You can't go wrong with clear, otherwise follow the color clues on page 23. Tip: tinted groomer will fill in minor bald spots.

- **WATERPROOF LIQUID BROW COLORS** are the hardest to master, but once you do, they offer the best results. Simply apply a little of this liquid corrector (it resembles liquid eyeliner) on the back of your hand and dip an angled liner brush into the color. Sweep onto the brows in little feathery strokes. Liquid brow color is perfect for humid climates and for women who have blonde, sparse, or missing brows. It will stay on all day.

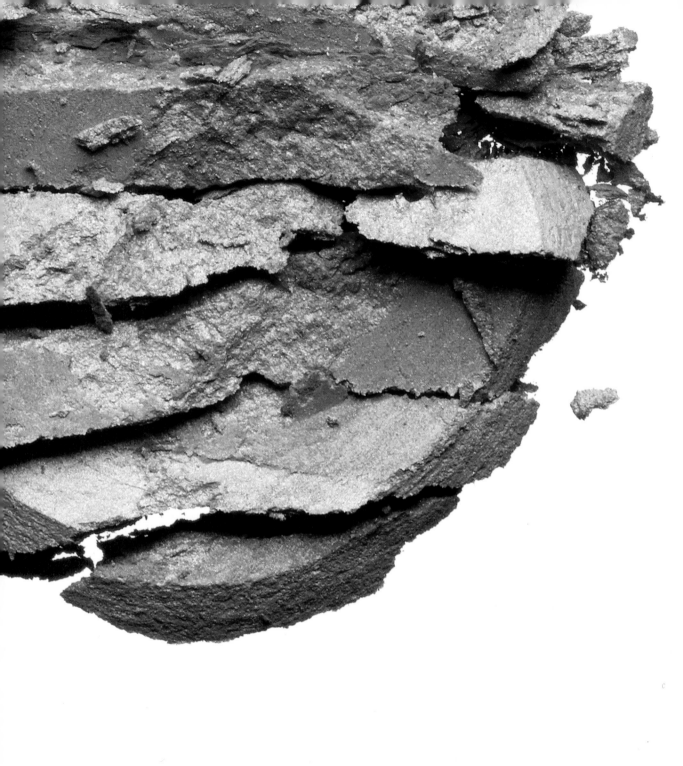

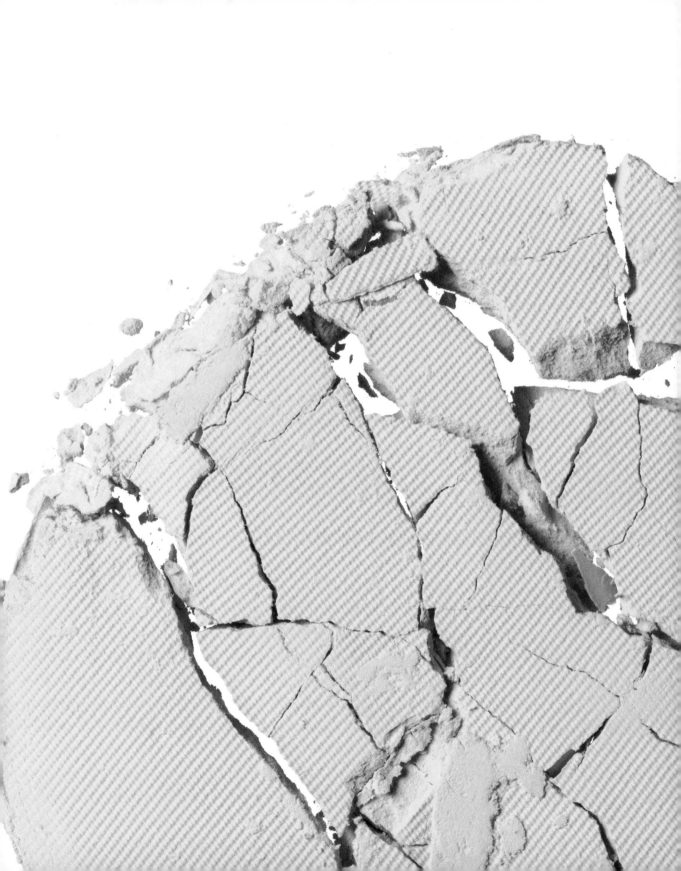

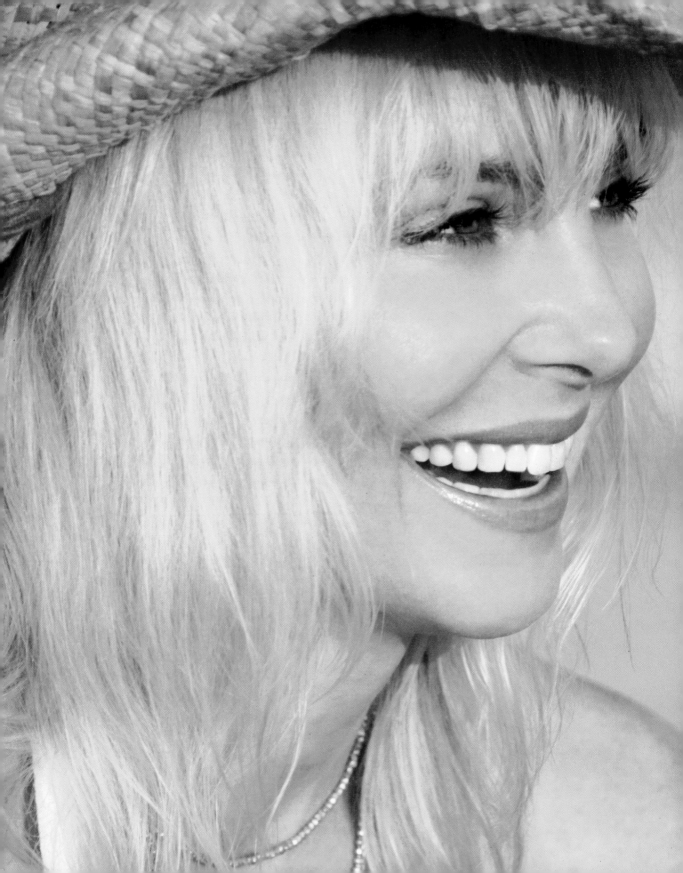

chapter three

FOUNDATION, CONCEALER, AND POWDER

A beautiful complexion (natural or achieved via the tips I give here) is like a canvas—it sets the stage for a more radiant you. When you get it right, your skin will glow; you'll look younger and your makeup will look better. Faking it doesn't require fancy tricks—if you make the right product choices.

FOUNDATION

Finding the perfect foundation can seem like a daunting task for any woman, no matter what her age or skin tone, but it is easier than you think. Foundation formulas have become so advanced that you should never feel like you're wearing a mask. Foundation should not be used to re-create your skin, but rather to enhance it.

Choosing the Right Shade

The right foundation color will disappear into your skin. To find the perfect shade, narrow down a selection of hues to the three closest matches of your skin color. Next, dab a stripe of each on your jaw, to see which one matches your skin exactly. You should look at the stripes in natural daylight—run outdoors, and peek into a mirrored compact. Note: I have found that some women with rosacea or sunspots may have a much darker skin tone in their face compared to that of their neck and chest. When this is the case, choose a color that falls in between the shades of your face and neck, smooth it in from your face down over your jaw, and feather it down your neck. This will ensure that everything blends together. Remember: always purchase foundation that you can either test before you buy or return if the color is wrong.

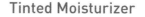

Tinted Moisturizer
Best for normal to dry skin that's naturally flawless. Tinted moisturizers contain a little bit of color that adds the barest coverage. These moisturizers are so sheer that they require little blending. Many also contain sunscreen, so you can cut out that extra step in the morning.

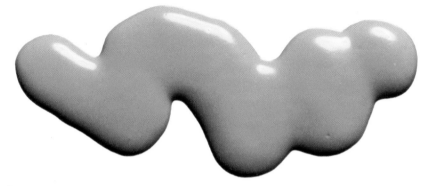

Liquid Foundation

Best for all skin types. This classic foundation offers a step up in coverage from that of tinted moisturizer. Liquid foundation feels light but helps downplay minor imperfections like tiny scars, acne, or unevenness. Available in oil-free, regular, hydrating, firming—whatever you need, it's out there. For more coverage, let it set for a minute, then add another layer where needed.

Cream Foundation

Best for older skin and dark skin tones. Liquid formulas can fade away on dark complexions or older skin that may need extra coverage, but because creams don't soak into skin, the pigments in cream foundations stay truer longer. This category of foundation includes creams, sticks, and cream-to-powder formulas. Since they are usually oil based they are a good option for very dry skins. Carefully blend in cream foundations so they don't look "thick" on your skin. Take your time and work in good light to ensure that you don't leave any demarcation lines.

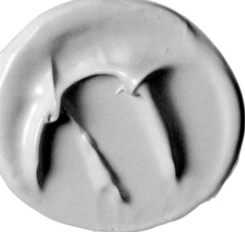

Mineral Powder Foundation

Best for sensitive skin. Mineral powder foundations get their coloring and full coverage from crushed natural earth minerals, such as zinc or iron oxides, and contain no chemical dyes, waxes, or preservatives, making them ideal for sensitive skin. You can swirl them on in layers for more coverage. They can be a bit chalky-looking on dry skin.

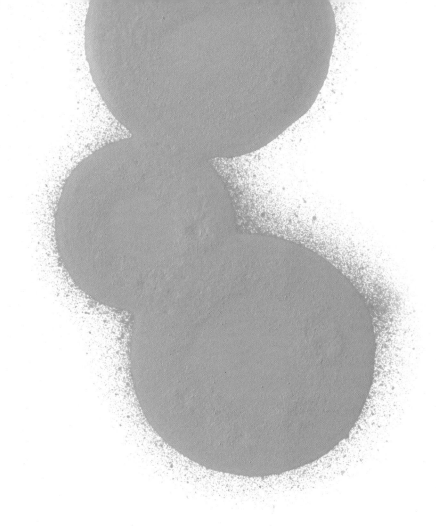

Aerosol Spray Foundations

Best for skin that needs a little extra coverage but with staying power. Aerosol spray foundations started as a makeup artist's trick (airbrushing body foundation onto bikini models for flawless results), and are now offered by some beauty brands for the face. The refined mist gives you a flawless crease-free coverage that lasts all day. You can control the amount of coverage by using different application techniques. For heavier coverage, spray directly onto the face. For a more sheer look, spray it on a sponge that has been dipped into a little moisturizer, then apply. This is one of my favorite ways to create perfect looking skin.

> **TOOLBOX: SPONGES.** Choose non-latex sponges—the ones with a smooth, pore-free surface that won't absorb (and waste) foundation. Sponges create an easy and flawless finish without getting your fingers all messy. Use one sponge every few days to keep foundation application nice and clean.

PREP SCHOOL

If your skin has a lot of oil, acne, or fine lines, you can apply certain products *under* foundation to boost its perfecting ability.

Foundation primer looks and feels like lightweight lotion. It helps foundation glide on smoothly and keeps it from seeping into pores or wrinkles. At the same time, foundation primer helps makeup last.

"Mattifyers" are serums or gels used to combat shine throughout the day. They can also be found as an ingredient in some oil-free moisturizers. I prefer to buy them on their own because you can target your T-zone, where greasiness is always a problem. This product controls shine all day (almost like a facial antiperspirant). Apply it to the areas that get the most greasy, let dry, then apply oil-free foundation.

Fast Fix

Tired? Look it? Mix a little liquid shimmer into a few drops of foundation for a fresh, awake glow.

Secret Weapon: Light Reflectors

A lot of foundations now come with ultrarefined light-reflecting particles, which act like tiny mirrors that bounce light around skin for a lit-from-within glow. These foundations lessen the appearance of fine lines and wrinkles. It's all smoke and mirrors—but take advantage of it!

Eye Shadow Base

This is like a concealer for lids. Eye shadow base evens skin and makes powder shadows last. Trust me, you don't need to spend money on one. Just apply foundation, then add a dusting of face powder on your lids before applying eye shadow. Same benefits, one less product to buy.

Spot Coverage

Most of us don't need an entire face full of foundation. Often, it's just the central part of the face that shows unevenness: under eyes, the nose, and the chin. Apply here and blend outward toward the cheeks. The perfect color match ensures seamless results.

CONCEALERS

You only need two concealers: one for under-eye circles and another for blemishes, scars, tiny veins, or brown spots caused by sun or age. The less concealer you use, the better the results.

Under-eye Concealer

With age, the delicate skin under the eyes becomes thinner and more translucent, exposing veins and making us look tired. What can I say? It happens to all of us, even models. Here's how to play down the wiped-out look.

Best formulas I prefer light-reflective concealer sticks or crayons because they are more natural looking than cream or liquid formulas. These will brighten the area instantly. If you find that a crayon is a little too dry, dab it on the back of your hand, mix in a tiny bit of liquid foundation, then apply to your skin with a concealer brush.

Best shades For the most natural results, use a formula one shade lighter than your foundation. If you have light skin, make sure that your concealer has a subtle pinkish cast; if you're olive, it should have pinky-beige undertones, and dark skinned women need a concealer in the golden-beige family—these colors will counteract the pesky blue tinge.

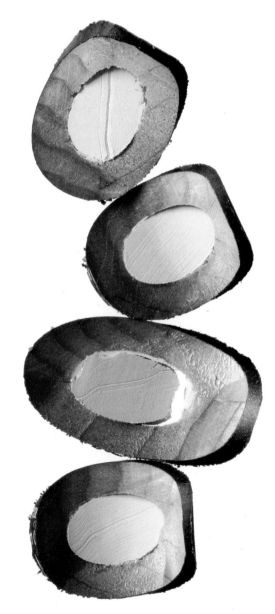

Fast Fix

For *extremely* dark under-eye circles, mix a little blemish concealer with your under-eye concealer for maximum coverage.

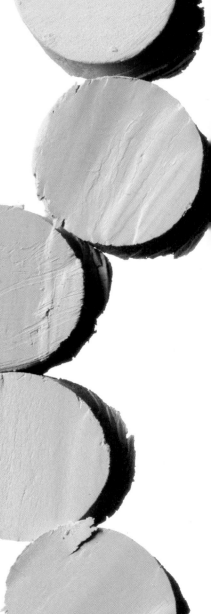

Concealer for Blemishes, Scars, Veins, and Sunspots

We all get blemishes from time to time, and a lot of us have more permanent imperfections we would like to conceal. With the right concealer your complextion will look flawless.

Best formula A creamy stick or pot concealer works great. It should be a little thicker than your regular foundation or it will slide off prematurely. If you're hiding acne, choose a concealer with pimple-fighting salicylic acid.

Best shade This concealer should match the color of your foundation, since the goal is for it to disappear onto your skin. *Avoid* concealers with green, yellow, or lavender hues; they never look right.

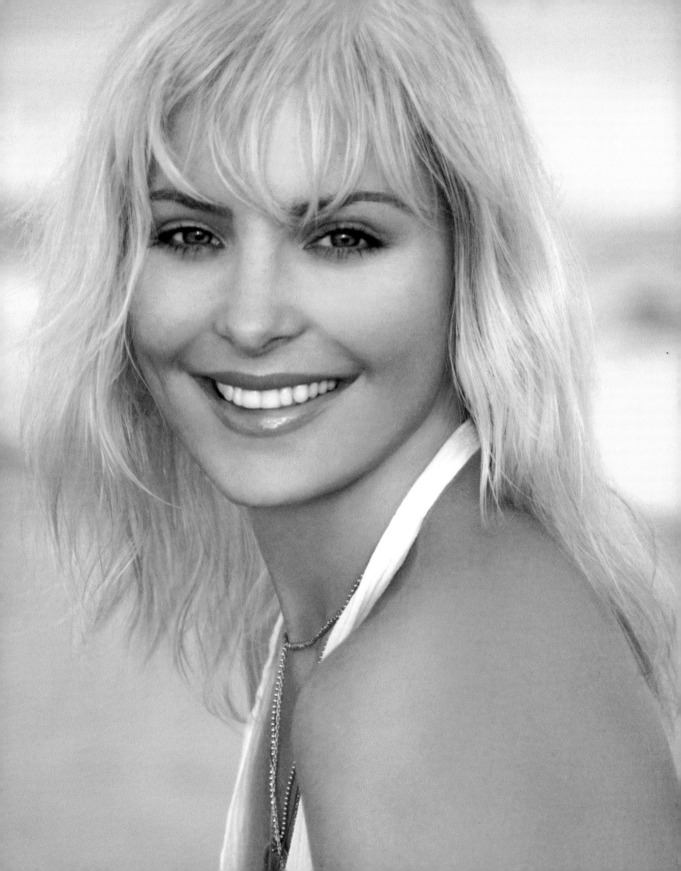

POWDER

Powder has two basic jobs: to eliminate shine and to "set" foundation and concealer so it stays put longer.

Best formula Don't buy heavily colored powder; it will add an extra layer of pigment you don't need and your skin will look too cakey as a result. Instead, use *translucent* powder. Although it may look like it has a nude tint in the packaging, it will appear colorless once applied to skin. Test in stores before buying. *Compact* powders are best because you can apply them using a powder brush or puff, and they will deliver less powder. Loose powders are harder to control. When you dip a puff or brush into them, the brush will pick up tons of powder and you will end up spending a lot of time shaking off powder to apply a tiny amount.

Fast Fix

Here's my favorite concealer trick of all time. If you don't want to invest in a separate spot concealer, dip your concealer brush into the leftover foundation that is a bit dried up in the cap. It's thicker than what's in the bottle and you can layer it on the spots.

Fast Fix

For an instant wake-up call, use a thin concealer brush and sweep on a little under-eye concealer from the outside of your lower lash line up to the end of your brow and blend. The concealer will highlight this area, and visually "lift" the eye. It works!

BLOTTING PAPERS

These little squares of paper mop up excess oil without removing makeup. They're perfect for shine control throughout the day. Avoid papers with powder in them—they can leave you looking dry.

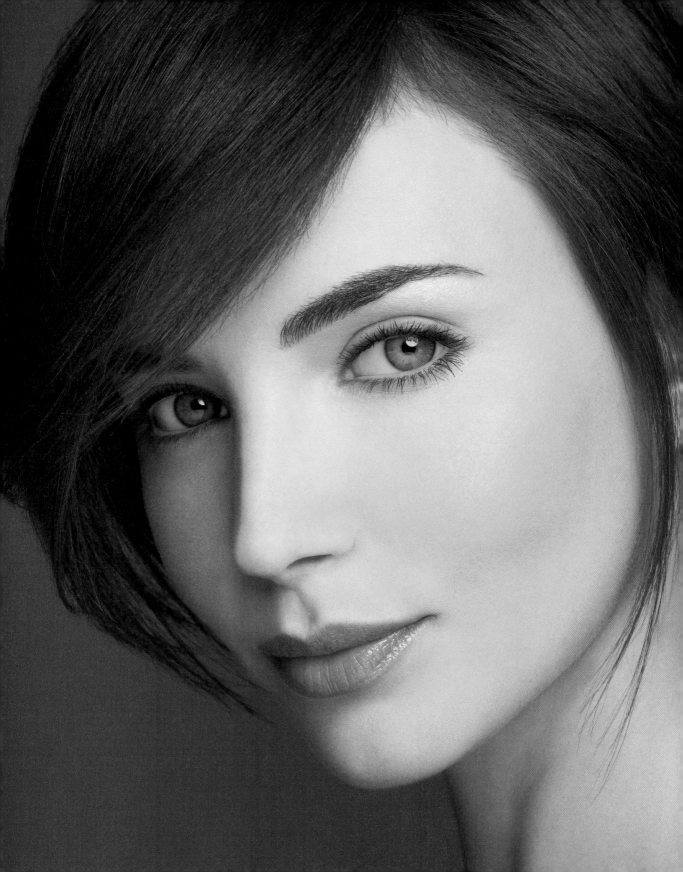

chapter four

THE 5-MINUTE FACE

Most women are intimidated by makeup. They don't have the time or the desire to take on a multistep routine, or they get scared by pushy makeup-counter salespeople who have their own commissions in mind, not a customer's best beauty interests. Women tell me all the time that they feel left out by beauty magazines whose focus has become celebrity beauty ideals and red carpet looks that don't relate to everyday life. In the end, many women adopt a *"Forget it!"* attitude. They throw on mascara and lip balm and run out the door, not feeling their best. But by following the steps of my 5-minute face, you can create a complete, polished makeup look without a hassle. It's what I use every day; it's fast—and easy!

THE 5-MINUTE PLAN

00:00–01:00   Smooth on foundation or tinted moisturizer

01:00–01:20   Pat concealer under your eyes with your ring finger

01:20–01:55   Spot conceal any redness from tiny veins or breakouts

01:55–02:15   Use powder to set your makeup

02:15–02:45   Sweep on highlighter

02:45–03:05   Apply blush

03:05–04:05   Line your lash line

04:05–04:50   Brush on mascara

04:50–05:00   Slick on lip color

THE STEP-BY-STEP BREAKDOWN

STEP 1: FOUNDATION **Application smarts:** Tinted moisturizer and foundation go on the same way: I prefer using a makeup sponge for blending—it makes the job go faster. Dip the sponge into a bit of foundation and blend over the face including eyelids and under the eyes. Lightly buff down the neck for a seamless finish. If some areas need more coverage, stipple on a second layer by using a light patting motion to push the foundation into the skin. This is a great technique to hide redness from rosacea without resorting to thick cover-up. Expect to use about a nickel-size amount for the entire face.

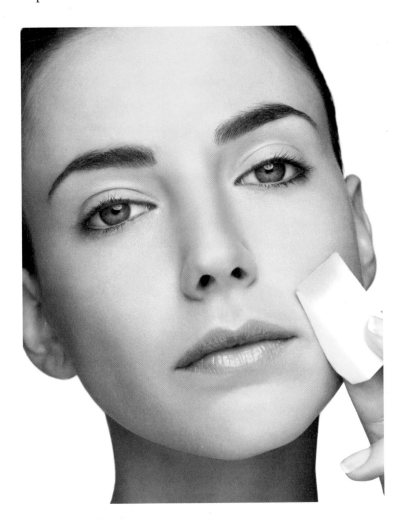

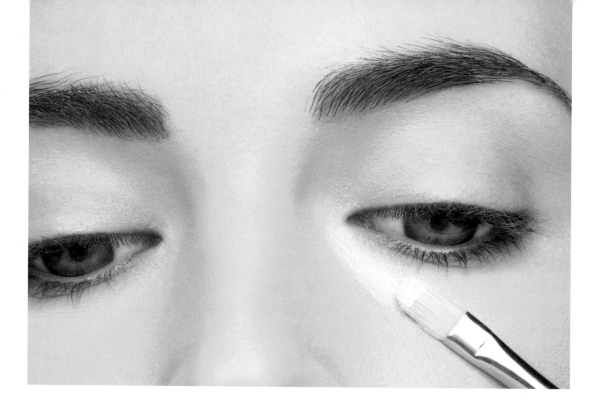

STEP 2: UNDER-EYE CONCEALER **Application smarts:** Since you've already applied your tinted moisturizer or foundation under your eyes, you'll need less concealer and will have a more natural finish. The most important thing to remember about concealer is less is more. If you load concealer on to obliterate a problem area, it takes on a dry, cakey look as the day goes on, and it will actually draw attention to what you're trying to hide! For *under eyes*, sweep concealer next to your eyes' inner corners (where dark color is most concentrated) and blend downward with a ring finger. Make sure to target only the dark areas of your skin; if you start spreading it up and down and all around you end up with that "I never took my sunglasses off on vacation" look.

Fast Fix

If you're bothered by your dark circles, shift the focus by playing up another feature, like your mouth. Wear bright gloss to draw attention from your under eyes.

STEP 3: SPOT CONCEALING **Application smarts:** For redness and blemishes, spot-apply concealer with a thin concealer brush. The bristles will be compact and tapered, and the thin tip allows you to "paint" concealer precisely where you need it. Afterward, use a finger to gently pat any edges, blending them seamlessly into skin.

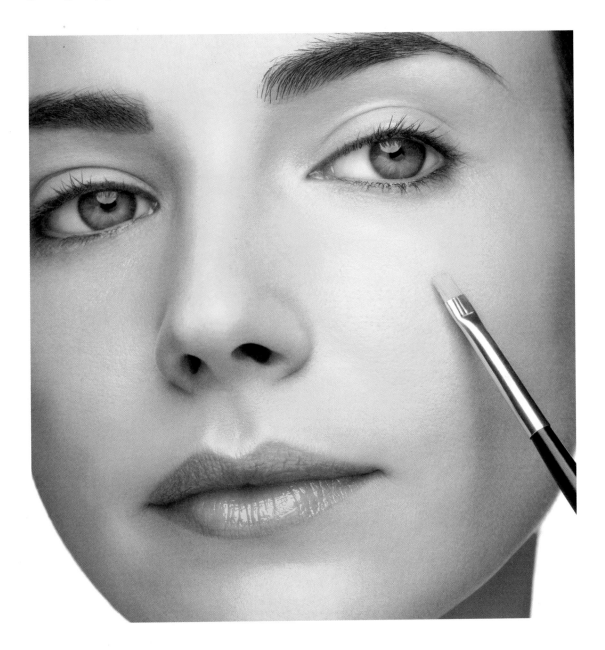

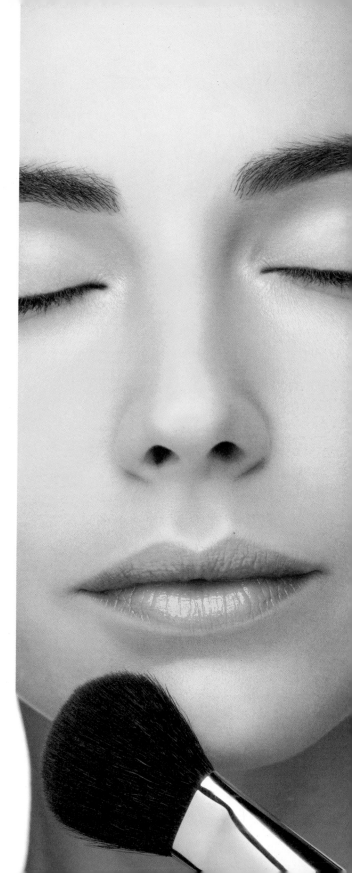

STEP 4: POWDER **Application smarts:**
Apply face powder with a clean *blush brush*. Yes, a blush brush: the smaller size makes it easier for you to target the few places where you need powder. In contrast, a classic puffy powder brush dusts powder all over, leaving skin looking overly matted. Less powder is modern and leaves skin dewier; dust it down your nose, across your chin, and over your cheeks and eyelids. That's all you need. A little can be applied under the eyes, but use only enough to set the makeup without causing it to cake together. I like to leave the tops of the cheekbones powder-free. Even if you have oily skin, having a bit of shine in this area gives you a youthful dewy look. If your skin is too matted down, you'll look dry and tired.

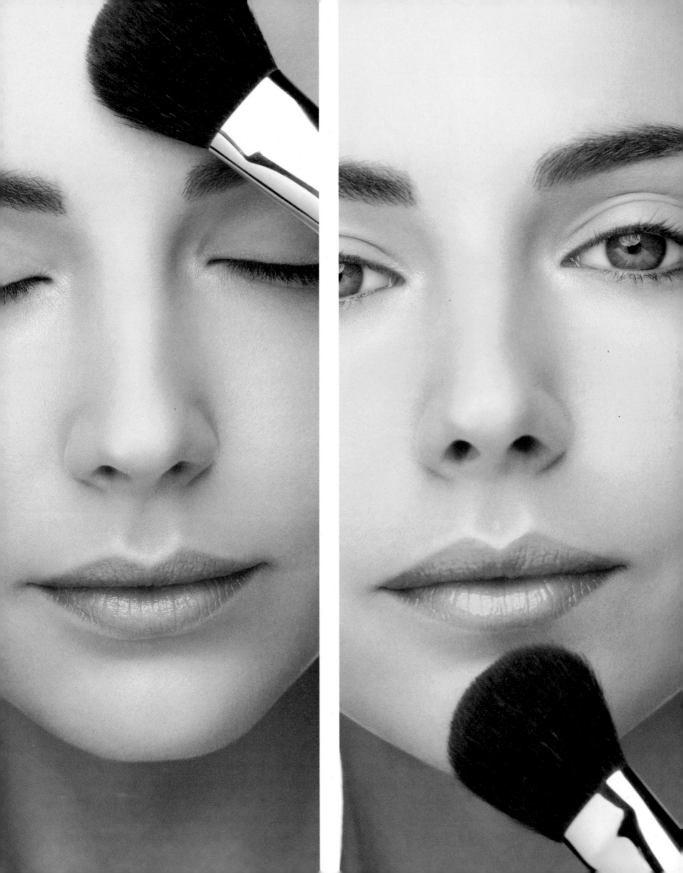

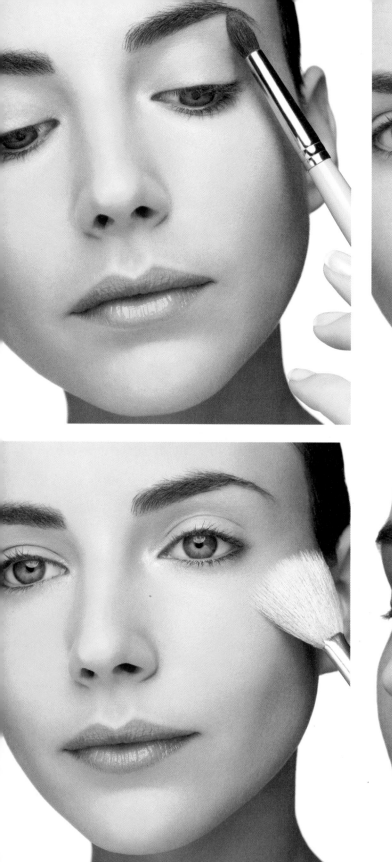
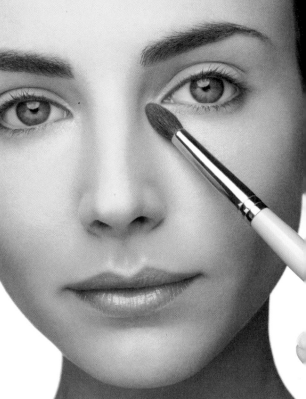
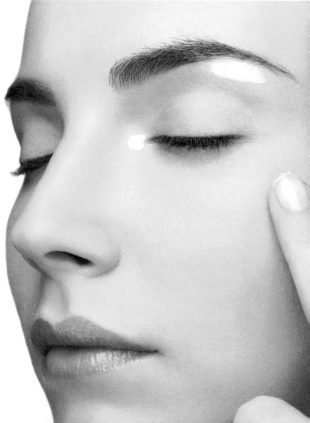

STEP 5: HIGHLIGHTER Highlighters are my secret weapon and the key to the 5-minute face. These pearly shimmers come in fine powders, sheer creams, luminizing liquids, or light-reflecting crayons and bring light to the face, blending into the skin to become almost unnoticeable—except for an ethereal gleam. Powders go on faster, so use one here to save time. After you apply it, tilt your face, you can see the tones of the color prisms, giving your face and eyes that luminous glow.

Application smarts: With an eyeshadow brush (or Q-tip), sweep on a little *powder highlighter* in three places: under your eyebrows, on the inside corners of your eyes by your tear ducts, and on top of your cheekbones (see box below on cheekbones). And for *cream or liquid highlighter*, use before powder and tap on a small amount, blending it into your skin with your ring finger. The combination surrounds your eyes with radiance and makes them shimmer—no eye shadow needed! It also draws light to the upper part of your face for an instant lift.

FIND YOUR CHEEKBONES!

The tops of your cheekbones are a key place to apply highlighter because it draws the eyes upward, highlights your bone structure, and gives the face more radiance. To find the top of your cheekbones, place two fingers side by side under the outer corner of your eye. That's the top of your cheekbone.

STEP 6: BLUSH Application smarts: Apply blush (one that mimics a natural flush) to the apples of your cheeks, which are the rounded areas that stand out when you smile very wide. *For powder blush,* apply using a brush made for face powder. Its large size will hug your apple and apply the color with a natural, seamless finish. *Cream blush* should be applied before face powder. It should be dotted on with clean fingers then smoothed in tiny circles until it looks like part of your skin. Add more dabs until you build up to the color intensity you want. No matter whether you use powder or cream, remember that you should look like you're blushing, not like you've been slapped in the face.

Fast Fix

BLUSH OVERLOAD! Applied too much blush? This will help: if you're dealing with a cream blush, take a makeup sponge, place a drop of foundation on it, and with tiny upward strokes, buff over your blush to soften the color. If you used powder blush, do the same with a *dry* sponge.

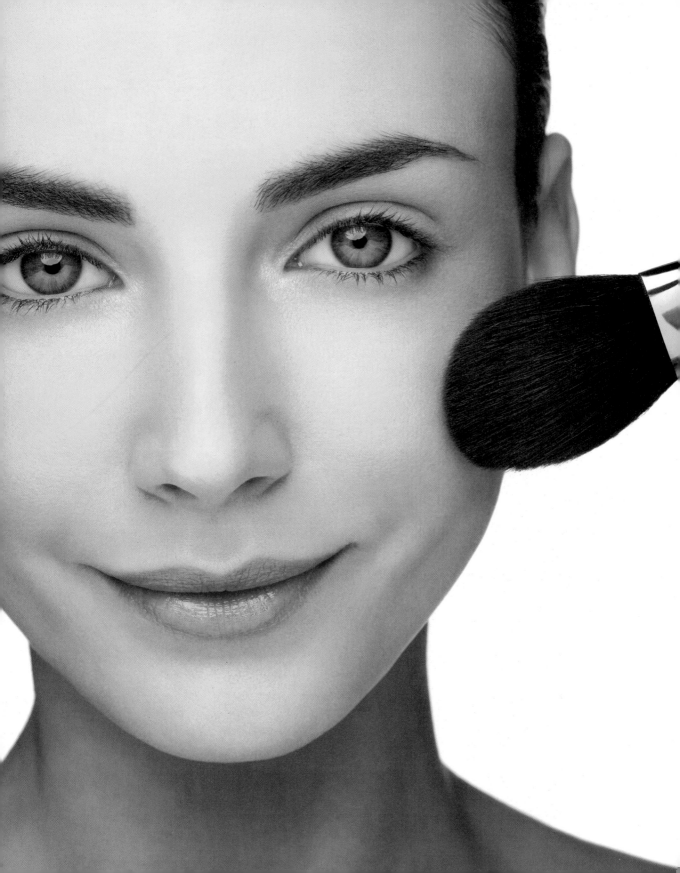

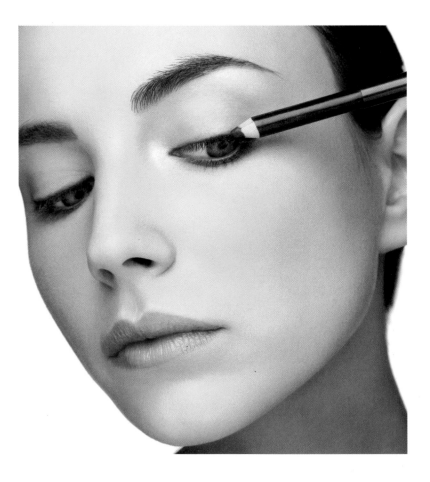

STEP 7: EYELINER **Application smarts:** Aim to apply eyeliner along your upper lash line as close to the roots as possible; wiggle the pencil using little back-and-forth motions to really work the color into the roots, then smudge with a Q-tip to soften the line. This will give the illusion of a thicker lash line, but your eyes won't scream "Eyeliner!" You can use whatever liner is left on the Q-tip to slightly smudge under your lower lashline for just a hint of color. Chocolate brown pencil liner is a universally flattering no-brainer shade. Cheap or pricey doesn't matter as long as it glides across skin without skipping, pulling, or crumbling.

STEP 8: MASCARA **Application smarts:** Tilt your head back slightly and look down to expose your lash root. Target the root as the first place the brush hits (it will deposit the most color there, which is where you want it), then glide the brush through to the tips. Apply one coat to your top lashes only. The bottoms are where smudges happen most and keeping them bare will save you potential cleanup time.

Fast Fix

I like black mascara on almost everyone. It makes more of a statement and gives you that extra *wow!* Keep an eye out for formulas with smaller brushes; they offer control for faster application and fewer clumps.

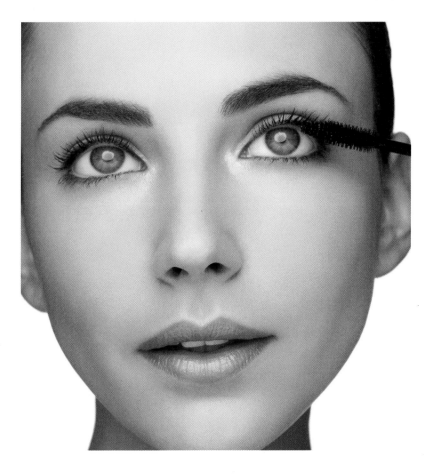

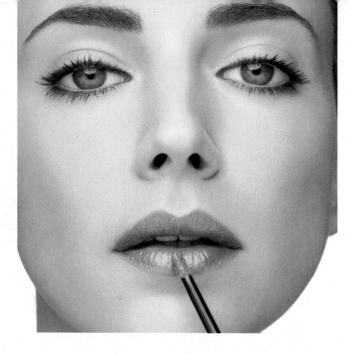

STEP 9: LIP COLOR **Application smarts:** The quickest way to add color to the lips is to use a tinted lip balm. This is a fast and natural way to add color, moisture, and protection in one easy swipe. Of course you can use your favorite lipstick or gloss. Cover your lips in color, then run a pinky finger over them to help "push" moisture and color into your lips.

CHECK YOUR LOOK IN THE MIRROR AND YOU'LL SEE—YOU'RE PERFECTLY polished in five minutes! Enjoy it, master it—and then see where else it can take you. Besides being the ultimate look for every day, my 5-minute face technique is the basis for all of the other (easy) looks covered in this book, such as one that's perfect for a black-tie event or one that makes you feel fantastic on a sexy Saturday-night date. You'll look and feel like a makeup expert, even if you aren't!

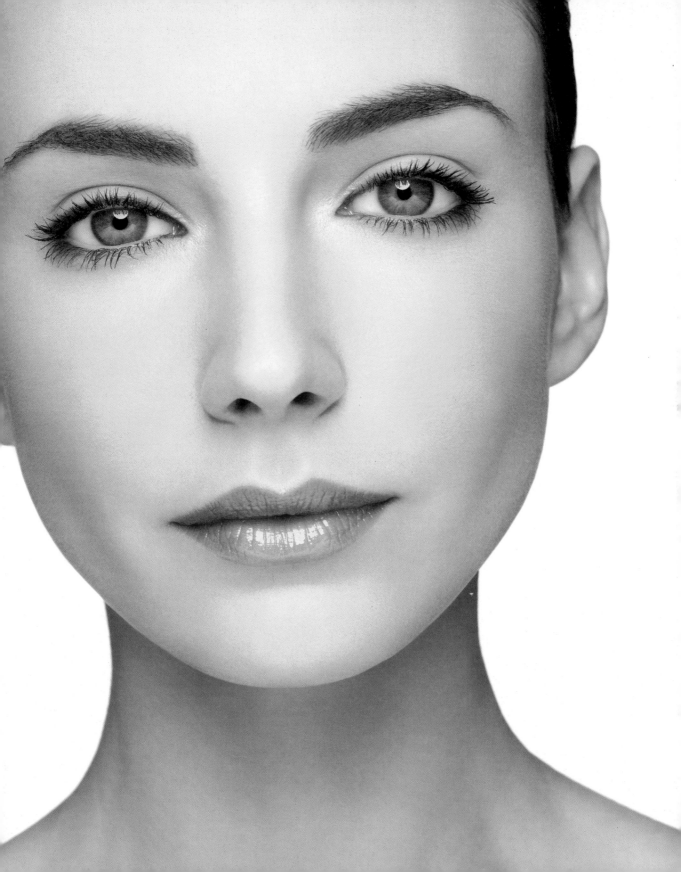

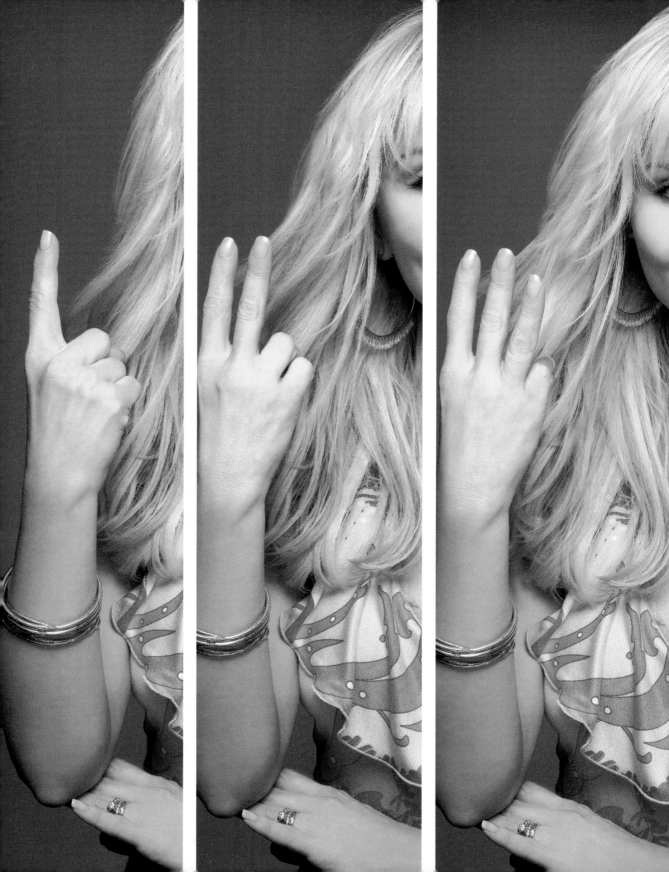

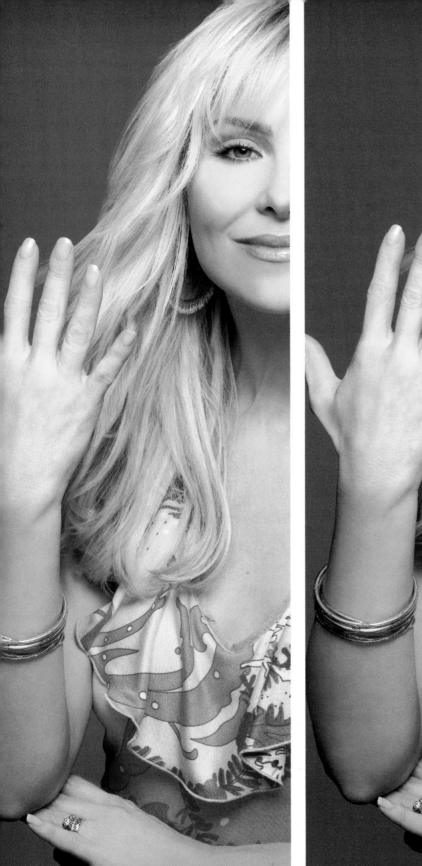
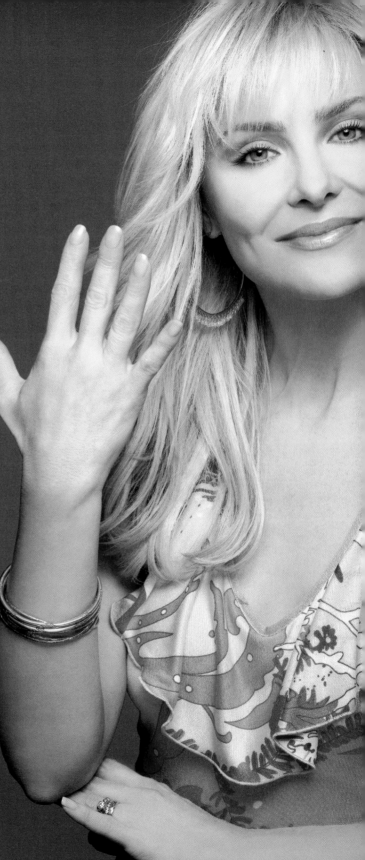

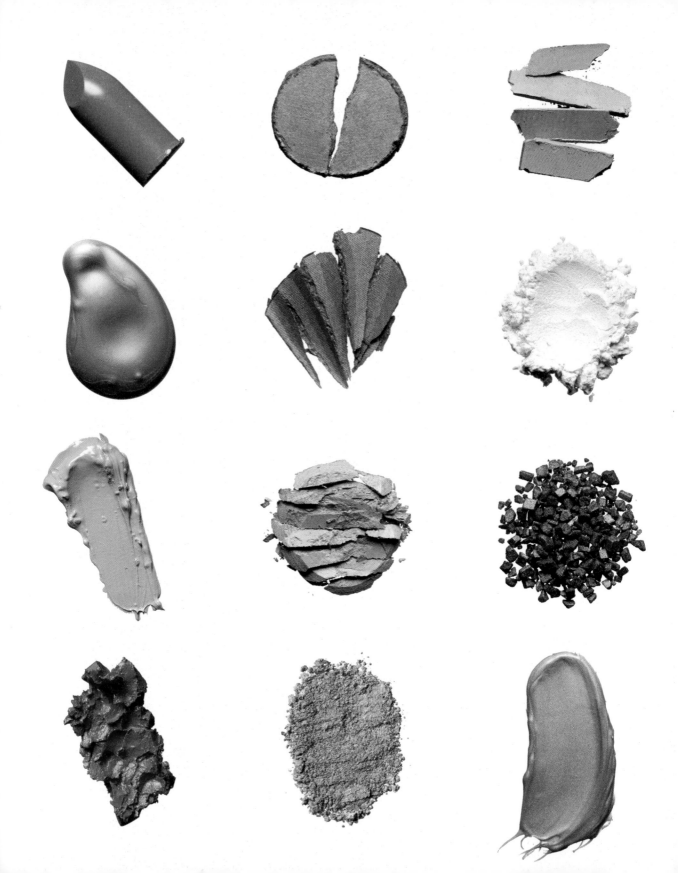

THE BEST MAKEUP COLORS FOR YOUR SKIN TONE

Beauty comes in all colors—it isn't one size fits all, and neither is makeup. What looks good on you may not work on someone else. When it comes to how to apply makeup, follow the 5-minute face steps or the looks in chapters 7 and 8, but use the chapter here as a general guide to choosing your basic, no-fail hues.

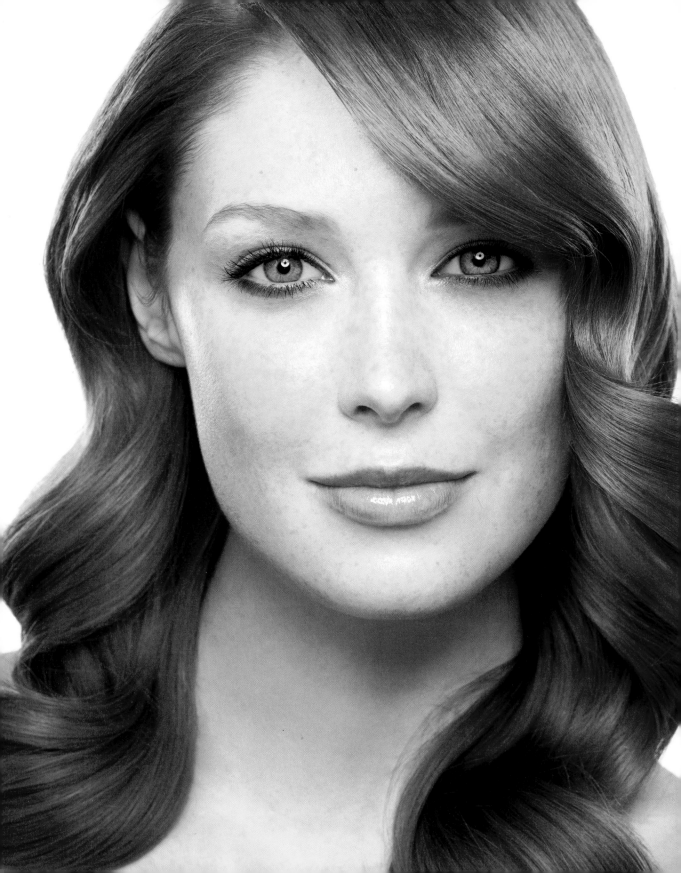

PORCELAIN-SKINNED REDHEAD

That romantic ideal of alabaster complexions is so alluring. I think of Botticcelli when it comes to these gorgeous women. Yet, a lot of women with this coloring have a tough time finding the makeup colors that look best on them. I blame the old mindset that cool pinks (like mauve) are *the* way to go for redheads. The opposite is true! Soft peaches, coppers, bronzy tones, everything your grandmother was told *not* to wear will make your skin glow (freckles included) like nothing else!

Highlight

Look for a sheer white or vanilla tone. Although you will barely see it, the effect will create a subtle "halo" of light that makes your eyes pop.

Eyes

Choose sable or chocolate browns, toasty taupes, pale golds, peaches, light bronzes, coppers, burgundy browns, eggplants, or khaki greens. Brown mascara looks more natural than black, which can be too harsh against fair skin; this is one of the few cases where I'll say this, otherwise, I prefer black mascara.

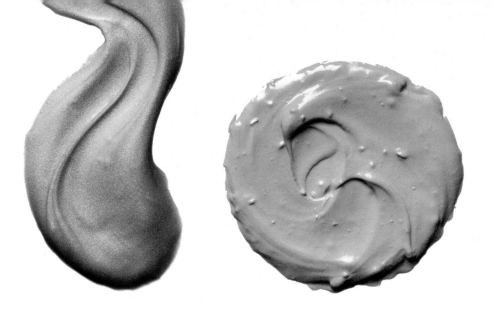

Cheeks

Pick peaches, apricot pinks, or light coral shades.

Lips

Think peaches and warm pinks, sheer corals, apricots, honey-colored nudes, raisins, and gold-flecked reds.

Fast Fix

Fair-skinned beauties with light-colored lashes, listen up: choose mascara with a shortish wand (about three-fourths of an inch long). It allows for more precision than do long or curved wands, so you can better reach those lighter lash roots. The best way to apply; wiggle the brush back and forth ever so slightly at the roots, then sweep up to the tips.

Beware the Invisible Brow Fuzzies

Who knows why, but if you are super fair, chances are that your brow bone is decorated with baby fine blonde hairs. You may barely notice them, but once you slide on highlighter, they'll show. Keep this in mind when you groom your brows—work in bright light (sunlight, ideally) and tweeze those tiny guys away.

SENSITIVE LIDS?

I find that a lot of women with this light coloring have sensitive lids, which become itchy or flaky after wearing shimmery eye shadow. Most likely, you're allergic to the mica that gives the glimmery effect. Skip shadow altogether and focus on highlighting under your eyebrows by blending in a pale white concealer under your arch. Next, smudge shimmer-free gel-formula eyeliner into the lash line and finish with hypoallergenic mascara. This will create all the definition and drama without any of the irritating side effects.

THE FRECKLE FACTOR

Women who have porcelain skin, especially redheads, tend to be blessed with freckles. People associate freckles with youth—a good thing! They give you a fresh, sun-kissed look. So please love your freckles and don't try to hide them behind concealer. Let them show!

BLONDES

Blondes come in a wide range of skin tones, from porcelain to olive. Colorful shades like pinks and rose bring color to the face and provide contrast.

Hightlight

My favorite shade for blondes is an opal irridescent shimmer. (Opal has a blue-pink oil-in-water glow that shows when light hits it.) It gives the skin a sexy, ethereal look.

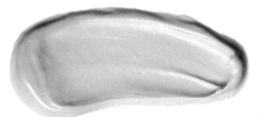

Eyes

Choose shades in cool browns, taupes, bronzes, granite, tawny pinks, pastels, mauves, and plums.

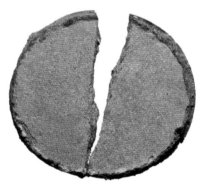

Fast Fix

Blondes tend to have eyelashes with blonde tips. If you're in a hurry, simply sweep mascara over the tips for quick, natural definition. For a more permanent fix, get your lashes tinted at a local salon. They use a vegetable dye that is perfectly safe for the eyes, and the color lasts about a month.

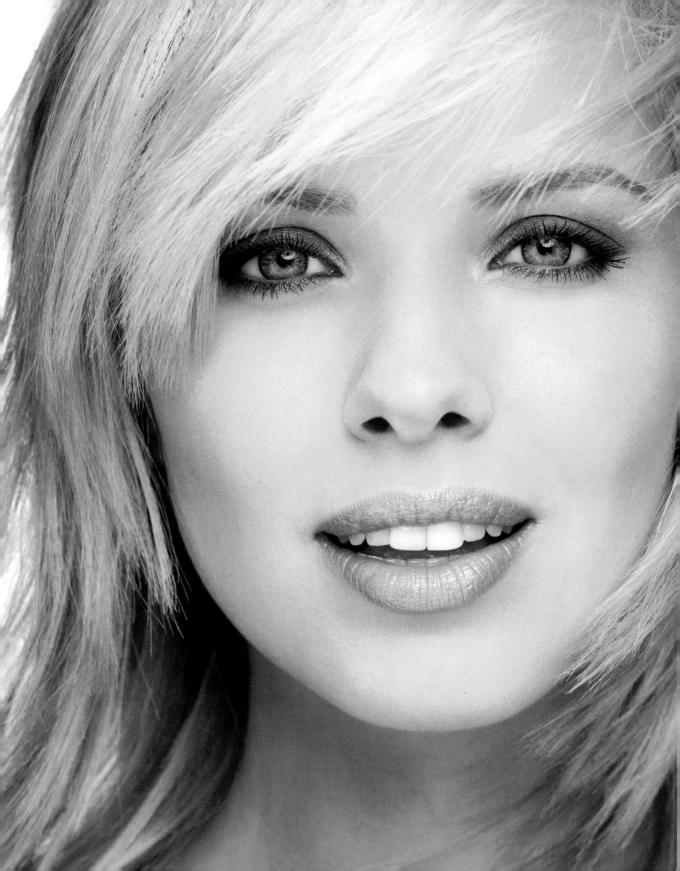

Cheeks

Roses, pinks, pinky bronzes, corals, and cool peaches all create a fresh and healthy look on blondes.

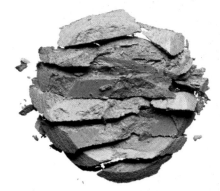

Lips

Think pink, mocha pinks, peachy pinks, sandy pinks, roses, mauves, golden raspberry, and cherry reds.

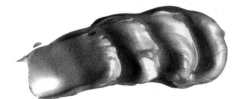

TIPS

- Light shimmery colors make lips look larger than darker ones.

- Plump lips by dabbing shimmery pale pink or gold gloss on the center of your lower lip.

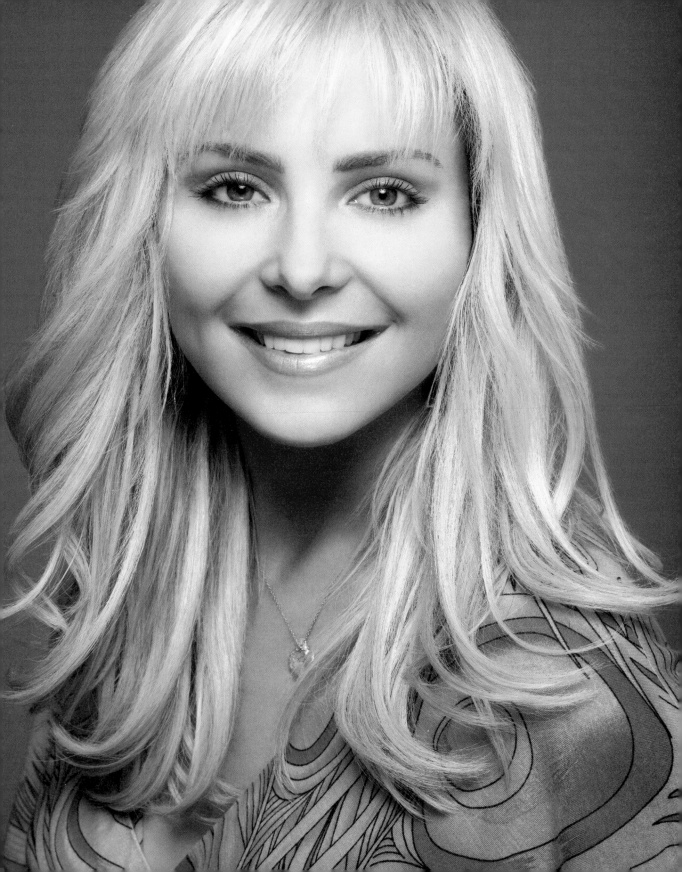

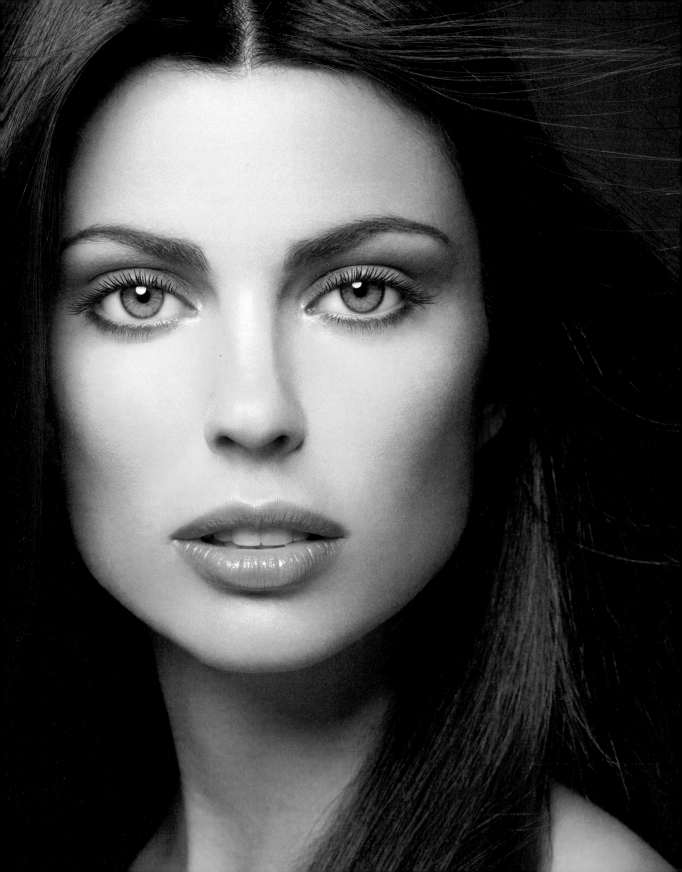

BRUNETTES

Brunettes have naturally dark eyebrows and lashes that frame and define their eyes, so they can get away with wearing less makeup. At the same time, their typically medium-toned skin allows them to choose from a wider range of colors than women with other skin tones.

Highlight

Champagne shimmer works best on you.

Eyes

Play with all shades of shimmering browns, silvery taupes, mochas, golden pinks, gold, bronze, navy and sapphire blues, purples and plums, burgundies, and forest greens.

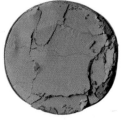

Cheeks

Choose rose, berries, bronzes, and terracottas.

Lips

Wear rose hues, berries, plums, bronzes, golden pinks, browny pinks, shimmering mochas, sheer corals, wines, and true reds. Avoid pastel lip colors (i.e., any shade that looks like it has white mixed in). These will just wash you out.

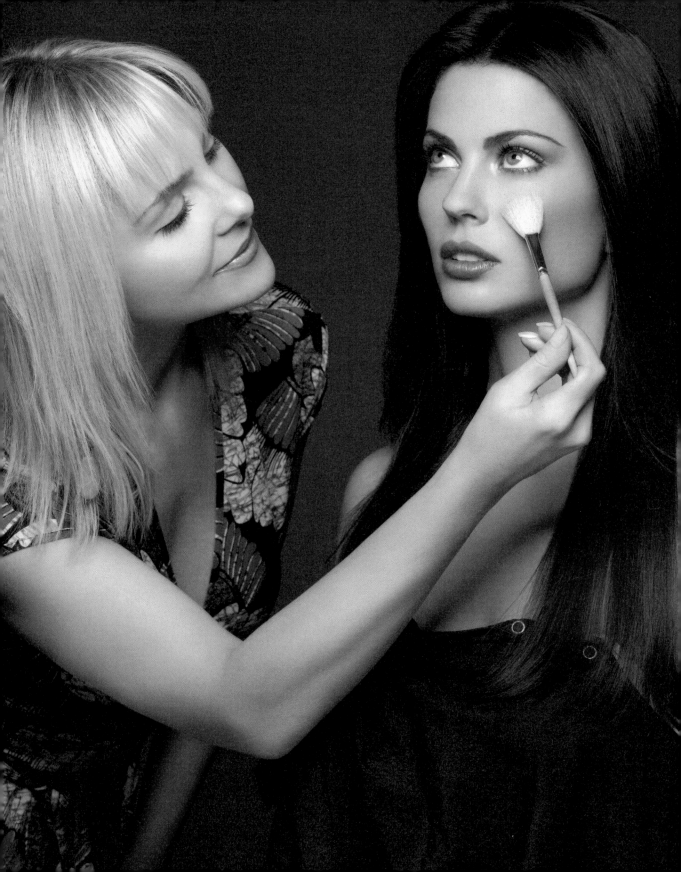

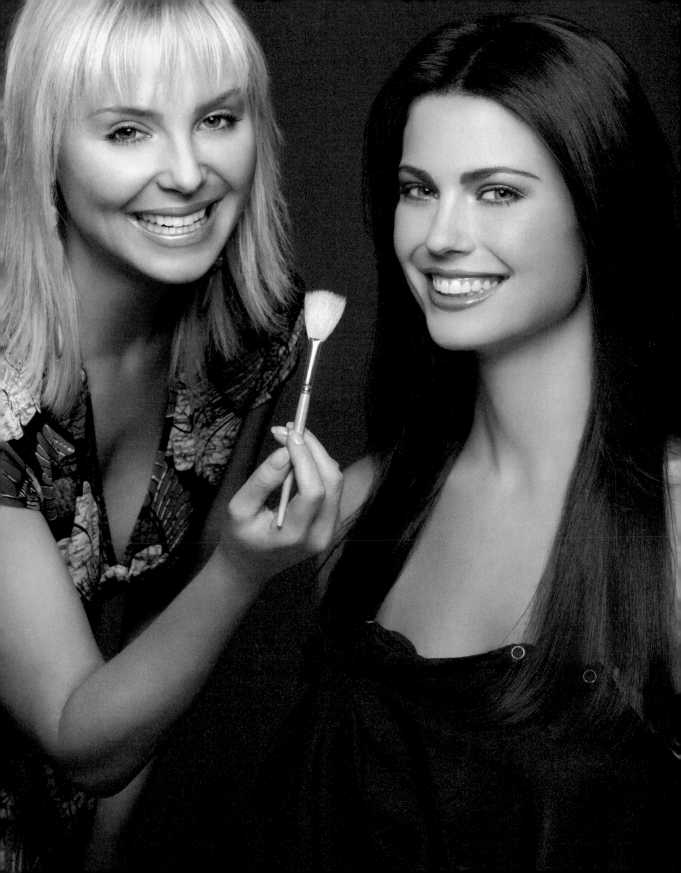

ASIAN

Asian women are among the most naturally beautiful in the world. They usually have full lips (the kind the rest of us dream of) and skin that never seems to age. Asian complexions looks best when color is brought to the cheeks and eyes are defined.

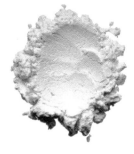

Highlight

Pale pink shimmer looks gorgeous and makes the most of your naturally beautiful skin.

Eyes

Choose colors in shades of tawny pinks, shimmering taupes and browns, burgundy, vanilla, emerald green, granite, silvery plums, and deep purples.

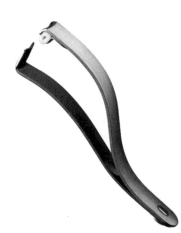

Fast Fix

Asian eyelashes tend to point downward, but if you curl them, you'll create an eye-opening effect. For best results, don't use a conventional lash curler that crimps your entire upper lash line at once. Instead, use a small, half-inch (or so) curler. It better allows you to follow your natural lash-line curve for beautiful results. Afterward, apply waterproof mascara, which will hold your curl longer than regular mascara.

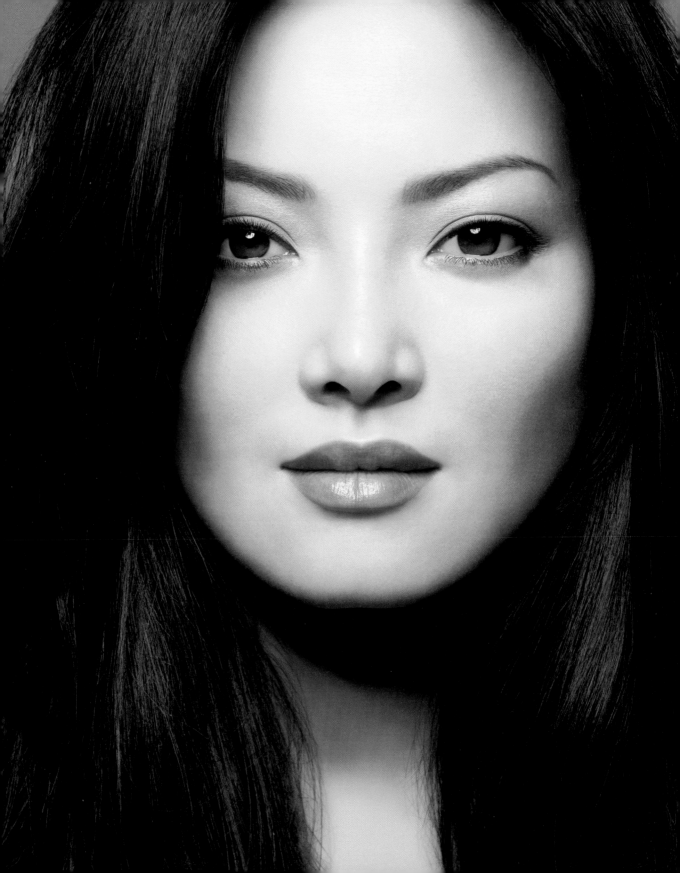

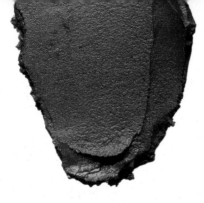

Cheeks

Wear pinks, berries, plums, and roses.

Fast Fix

Save time by turning a cream blush into a two-in-one product. Blend the cream blush on the apples of your cheeks then dab the same color onto your lips for a quick natural look.

Lips

Opt for pinks, like raspberry, roses, golden pink shimmers, pinky browns, mauves, deep plum stains, shimmering beiges, and nudes.

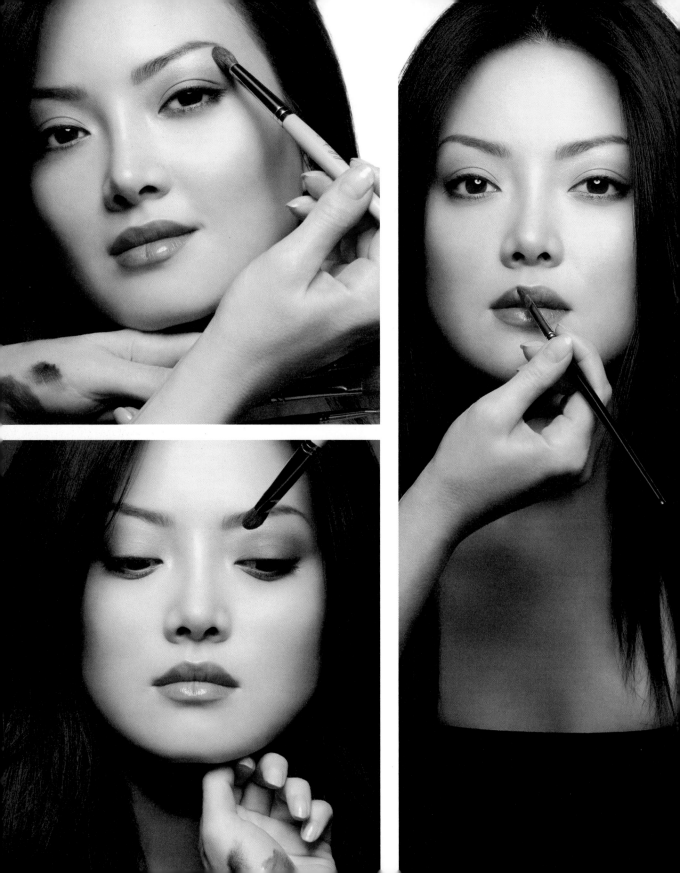

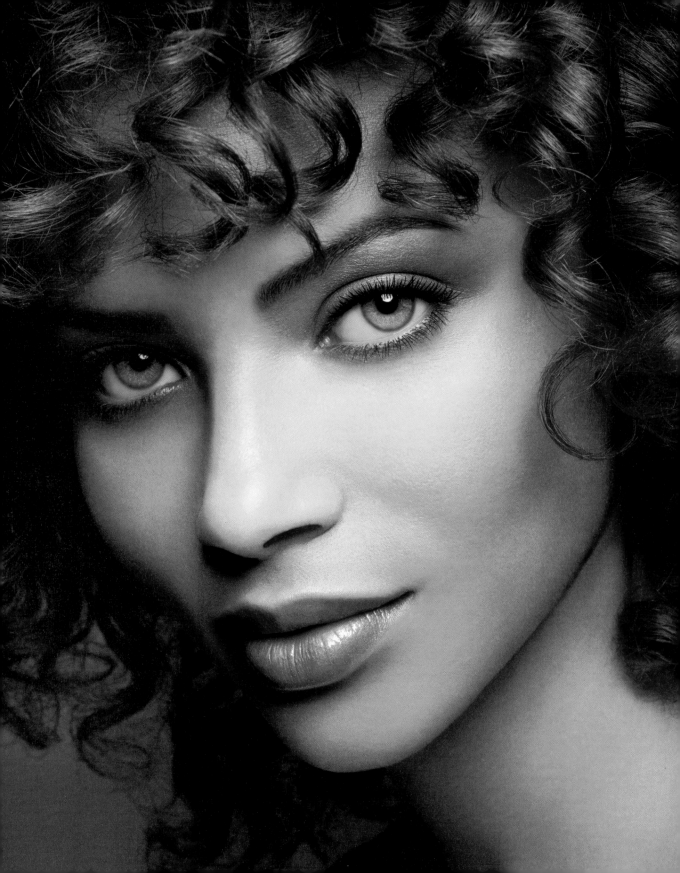

MOCHA SKIN

Women with this coloring have so many makeup hues to choose from, and they look especially radiant in golden colors.

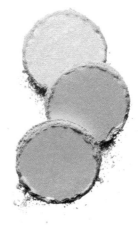

Highlight

Choose golden-pink shimmer. It will bring out the natural gold in your skin.

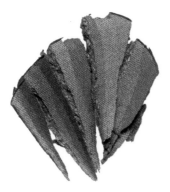

Eyes

Pick caramels, toffees, coffees, chocolate browns, deep wines, navy blues, granites, golds, bronzes, emerald greens, teals, deep plums, and violets.

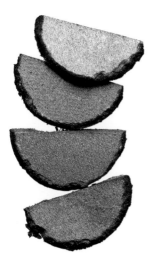

Fast Fix

You're usually blessed with lashes that have a natural curl. The upside is that you won't need a lash curler, but the downside is that when you apply mascara, your wet lashes bonk against your brow bone and leave tiny splotches. Avoid this by lightly wiping the wand with a paper towel before applying color. Then, sweep the wand back and forth vertically across the lashes as you apply. You'll see fewer smears.

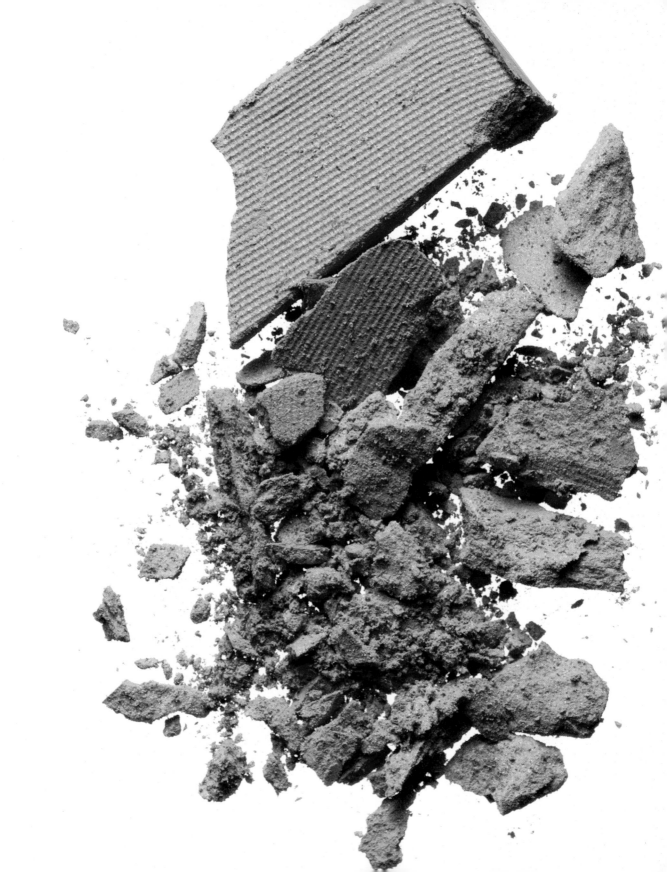

Cheeks

Look for berries, golden corals, bronzes, terracottas, deep warm pinks, and dark apricots.

Lips

Think sheer golds, beiges, coffees, caramels, toffees, bronzes, berries, plums, wines, pinks, corals, sheer raisins, and garnet reds.

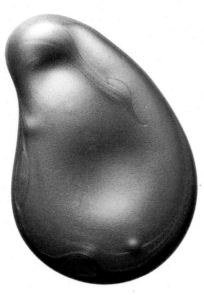

DARK SKIN

You can pull off bold, jewel-toned colors like no one else! Anything too light or sheer might look ashy.

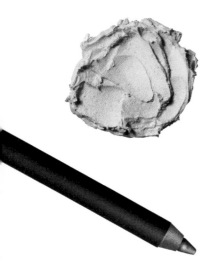

Highlight

Choose a true gold color. It's the perfect hue for you.

Eyes

Choose golds, coppers, bronzes, coffees, deep navy and cobalt, rich dark eggplant and purples, deep jewel-toned greens, slate and dark charcoal grays, metallics, ebony, and deep mahogany and chocolate browns.

Fast Fix

Make the whites of your eyes pop by applying sapphire blue pencil along the inner rims.

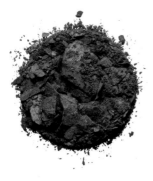

Cheeks

Think dark raisins, burnt orange, magentas, fuchsia (don't be scared, it will look beautiful on dark skin), and rich blood reds.

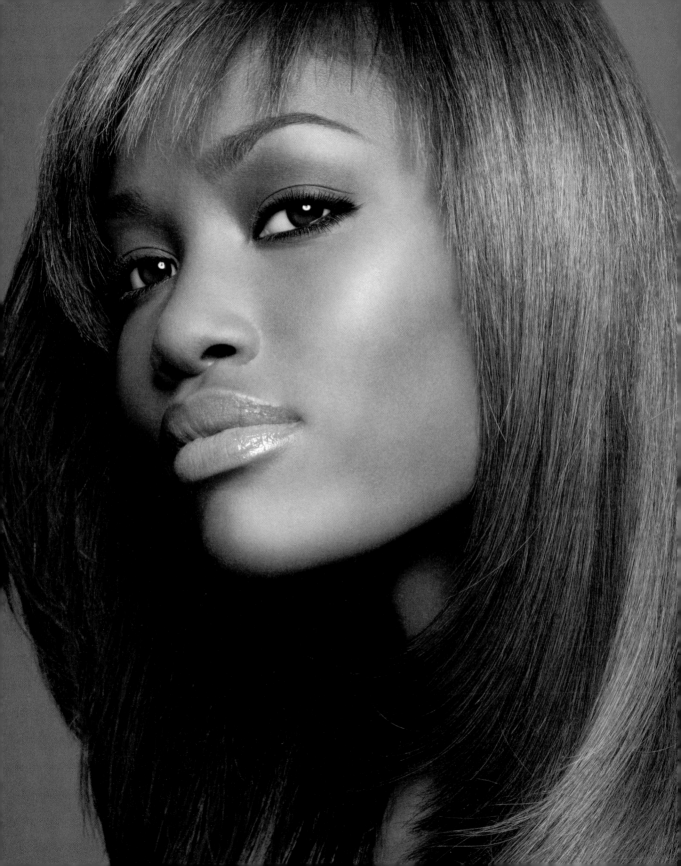

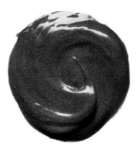

Lips

Pick sheer lip gloss in shimmery clears, golds, honeys, caramels, oranges, corals, tangerine, deep plums, bronzes, and bronzy pinks. Or choose lipsticks in sheer mahogany, blackberry, maroon, raisin, and deep red.

Fast Fix

Have curly brow hairs? Chances are, you do. Keep them smooth and in place with clear brow gel.

AVOIDING ASHINESS

I find that a lot of women with the darkest skin tones don't know where to turn when it comes to choosing the right foundation, concealer, or powder. If you pick the wrong product, your skin can take on a dull gray, ashy look. This happens because most beauty brands add too much pink pigment to their products, which turn grayish after a few hours. The best ones for you have golden tones in them, which stay true because they are more in sync with your natural color. Choose cream foundation and concealer; these will have enough pigment to stand up to your skin coloring. For powder, choose a darker tinted translucent. Throughout the day, zap oil with powder-free blotting papers.

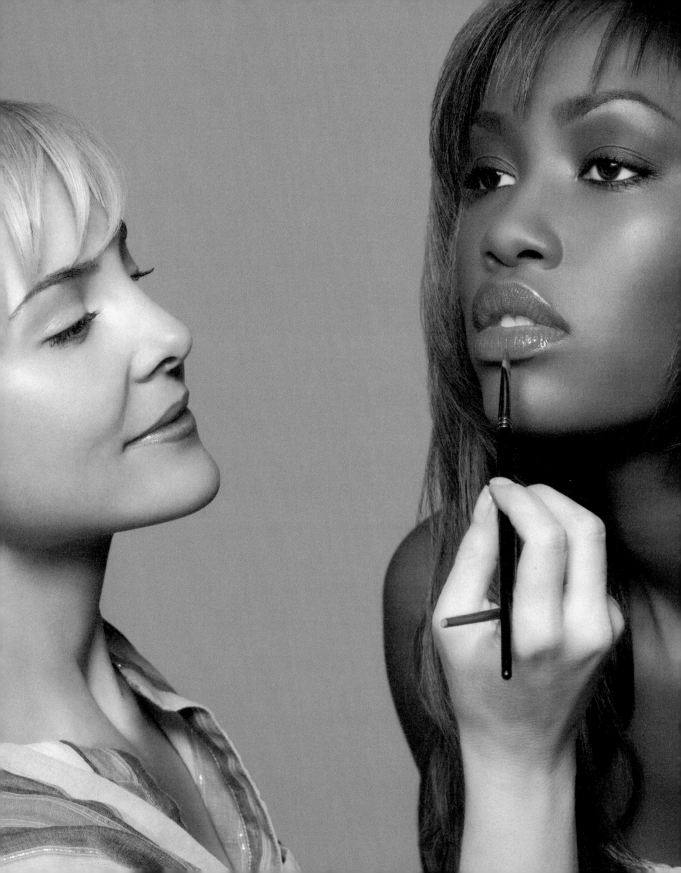

OLIVE SKIN

In addition to women with Hispanic roots, this group includes all women with olive skin, such as those from Italy, India, or the Middle East. Bright colors, like coral, on cheeks and lips, and everything from shimmery bronzes and pale golds to deep greens and blues around your eyes will play up your amazing skin color.

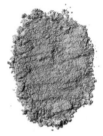

Highlight

I love pale golds and pinky golds to highlight the skin and create a luminous glow.

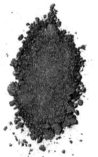

Eyes

Eyes look amazing in rich sparkling browns and burgundies, copper, bronze, gold, warm tawny pinks, eggplants and warm plums, deep forest greens, and sapphire blues.

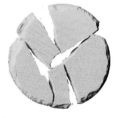

Cheeks

Think warm pinks, corals, brownish rose, apricot, and bronze.

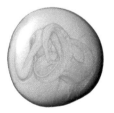

Lips

Go for warm pinks, sheer shimmery nudes, corals, peachy apricot, bronze and golds, golden berry shimmer, and sheer blood reds.

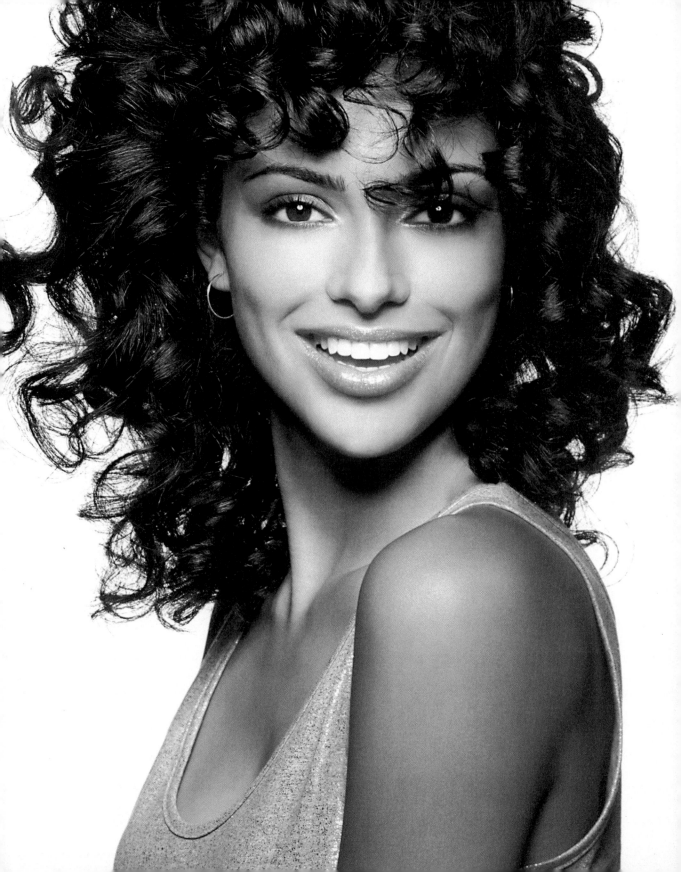

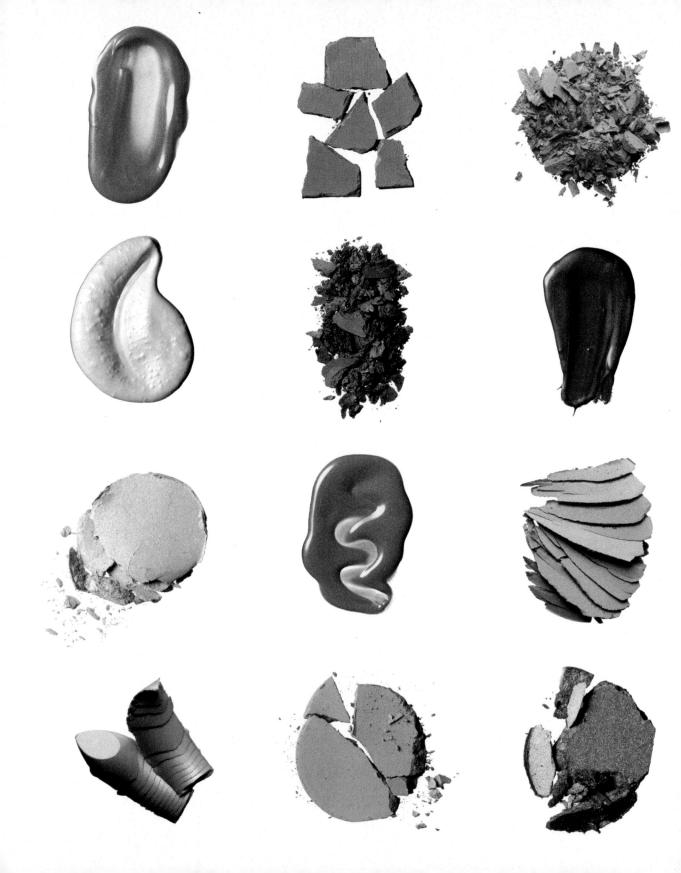

chapter six

BEAUTIFUL AT EVERY AGE

As we age, we go through subtle (and some not-so-subtle) changes that merit a color or texture tweak here and there to keep us looking our best.

TEENS

Girls just wanna have fun! And you can have so much of it playing with makeup because you can get away with a lot more at this age. This is not the time to be heavy-handed—your skin is glowing and alive, so don't hide it! Best strategy: play up one facial feature with bright sheer colors, then flirt away!

Skin Savers

In your teens, you're prone to breakouts more than at any other time in your life due to hormonal changes. Treat them with a solid routine: wash skin morning and night religiously and spot-treat breakouts with salicylic acid gels. Skip toners, which can be too drying. But do use oil-free SPF 15 moisturizer daily. Sunscreen is as important as everything else in your beauty routine, and if you make it a habit now, you will thank yourself in your twenties, thirties, and beyond.

$$$

You don't need to spend a lot of money on makeup when you're young. This is the time to experiment with shades that are "you," and do so with cheap drugstore offerings. When you start to hone in on the shades you love, invest in pricier brands that may have formulas that smooth on easier or last longer. Toolwise, have Q-tips on hand and use them to soften harsh edges.

Shimmery Colorful Eyes

Play with sheer washes of cream eye shadows in bright colors, or have a blast with glitter across your entire lid. Pass on dark eyeliner like black or navy, which looks overly harsh. Instead, opt for purples, teal blues or greens, and always smudge them into your lash line for a soft look.

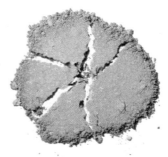

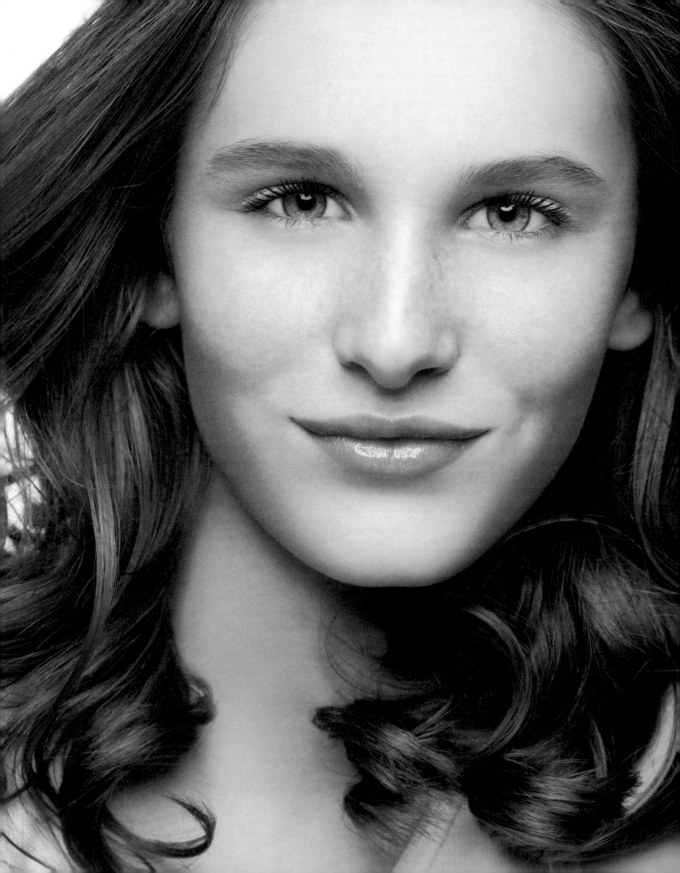

Colored Mascara

Just say yes! I love colored mascara on teens. Choose shades that match your eyes to really show them off.

Pretty in Pink

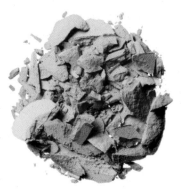

Most teens look beautiful in shades of pink. Wearing a bright sheer pink lip gloss and blush is a great way to accentuate your youthful rosy coloring.

Flawless Faces

You don't want to cover your fresh radiant skin with a lot of foundation. Instead, spot-conceal any breakouts with concealer (apply with a tiny brush for best results) and control shine with mattifying gels.

Danger Zone

Never ever share eyeliners, mascara, or lip products. Ever hear of pink eye or cold sores? These are highly contagious and are often transferred by sharing makeup.

Body Glitter

Take it easy and save it for a date or a dance. If you use it, go easy on the rest of your makeup, so you don't look like a Christmas tree ornament!

Chill out with the Tweezers

I have seen rampant overplucking on teens, and it's important to understand that brows may not grow back. All you need now is to tweeze any strays in between the unibrow area and ones that are obviously out of place on the brow bone. As for creating a new shape—it's not necessary.

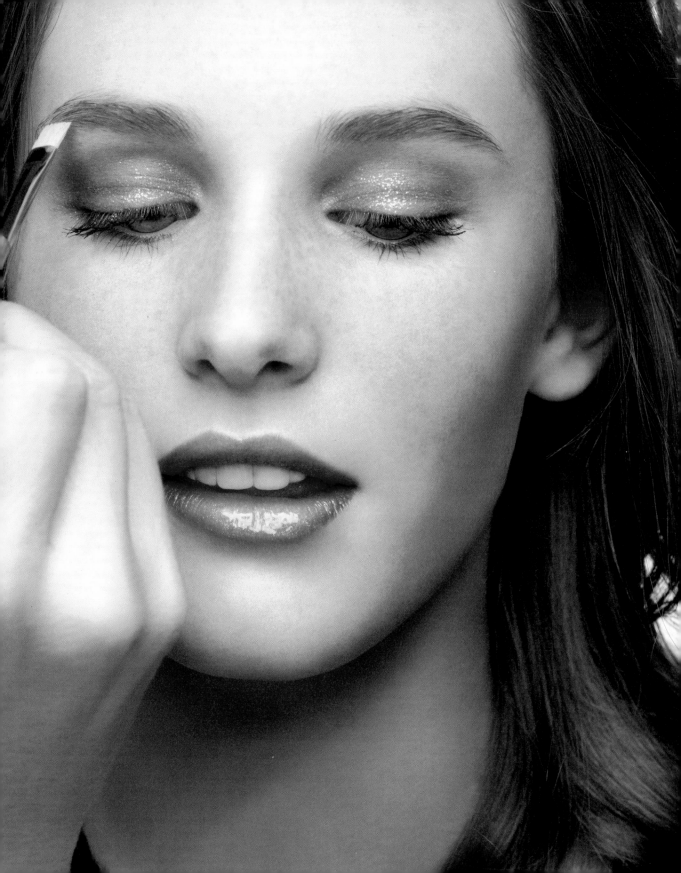

TWENTIES

This is the time to begin to discover your "look." During your twenties you can find the shades and styles that work best for you. You're probably going out on the town a lot, which means that you have more opportunities to test different makeup looks and see how you feel in them. Keep applying SPF 15 sunscreen daily. It's the easiest, cheapest way to put off skin discoloration, lines, and other changes for decades.

Go for a Glow

Fake a sun-kissed look with self-tanner. Play it up more by applying a sheer powder bronze to your temples and along your cheekbones. Use a light hand—if you overdo it, your skin will look "dirty." You want people to say, "Where'd you go on vacation?" not "What happened to *you*?"

Hot Date?

Don't think bold lip color, think smoldery, smoky eyes. Studies show that when it comes to makeup, most men hate thick, bold lipstick and prefer sexy, alluring eyes. Focus on creating a sexy, smoky eye and slick lips with a bare but shimmery, kissable color. If you're a gloss fan, blot it down. No one wants to smooch goopy lips.

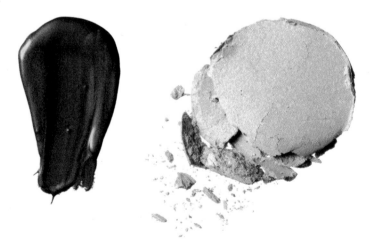

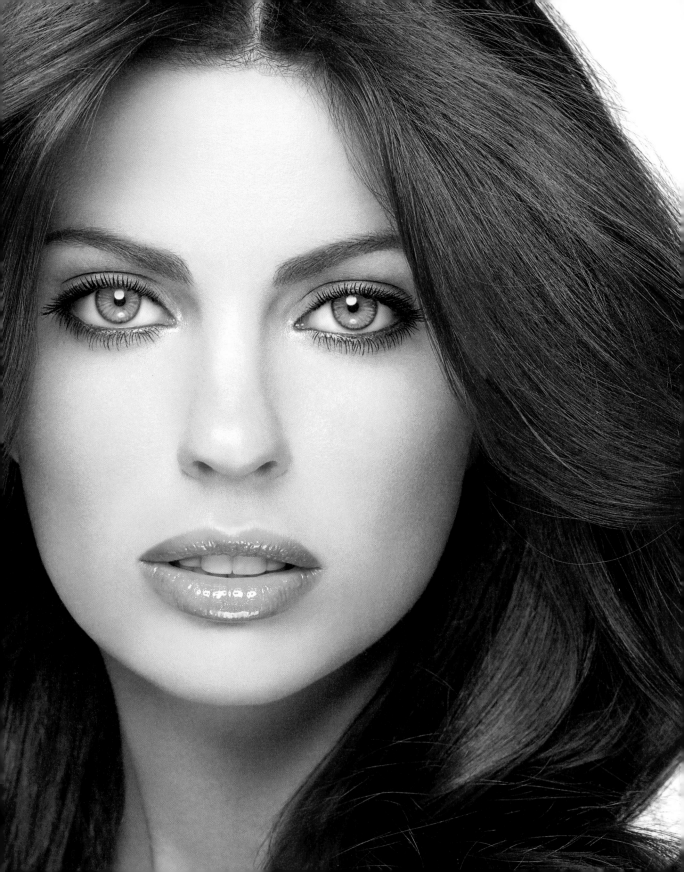

Fast Fix

GREASY CREASY. Do your eyelids get really oily throughout the day and cause your eye shadow to fade and crease? Before starting the 5-minute face, prep your lids with a little mattifying gel. This will make the colors you apply on top stay true longer.

Gloss Masters

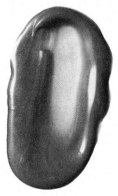

Your lips are naturally the fullest they'll ever be, so play them up with a luscious glossy finish. Wear gloss alone or over lipstick or lip stain. My favorite lip colors for twentysomethings are ripe shades, such as sparkling berries or sunny corals.

411 for Morning Puffiness

Overdid it last night, and now dealing with bags and puffy eyes? The key to depuffing is water. Drink tons of it for the rest of the day and use the good old fix of cold cucumber slices or cold, wet chamomile tea bags to soothe swelling. Keep the following tips in mind the next time you go out for cocktails—they'll help prevent puff: drink water before bed. Store firming eye gel in your fridge and use it when you wake up. Apply the gel, then cover your eyes with a cold washcloth and rest. The washcloth helps the gel sink in and acts like a cold compress to shrink the swelling.

Show Yourself

I find that some women in their twenties are still a bit insecure with their looks; they hide behind too much makeup or copy the style of their favorite celebrity. Honey, you're the star! Take a look at yourself and love what you see! Play with colors and trends that work best for you, but adapt them to accentuate your best features, your skin coloring, and your personal style. Let yourself show through!

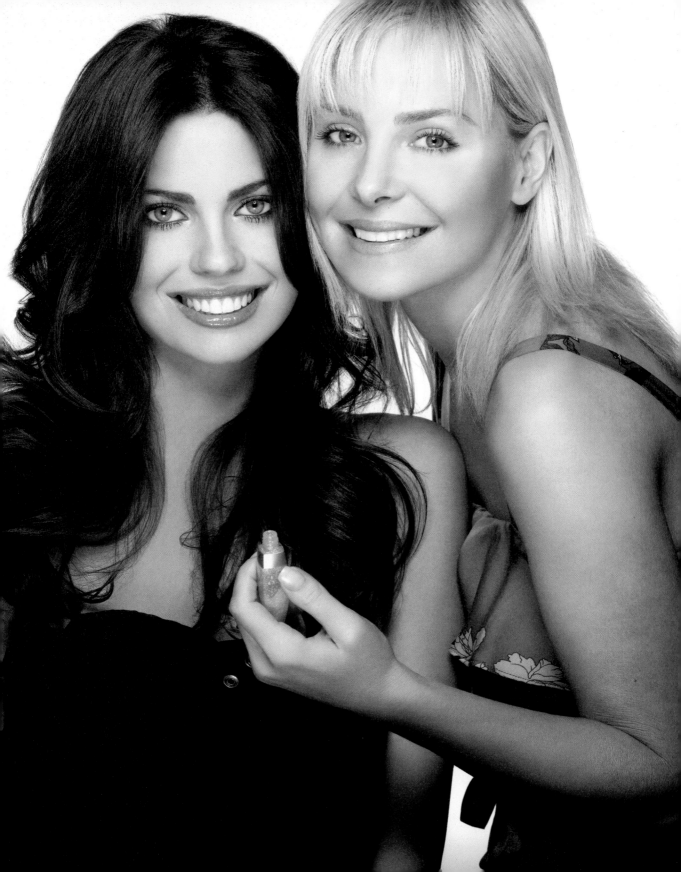

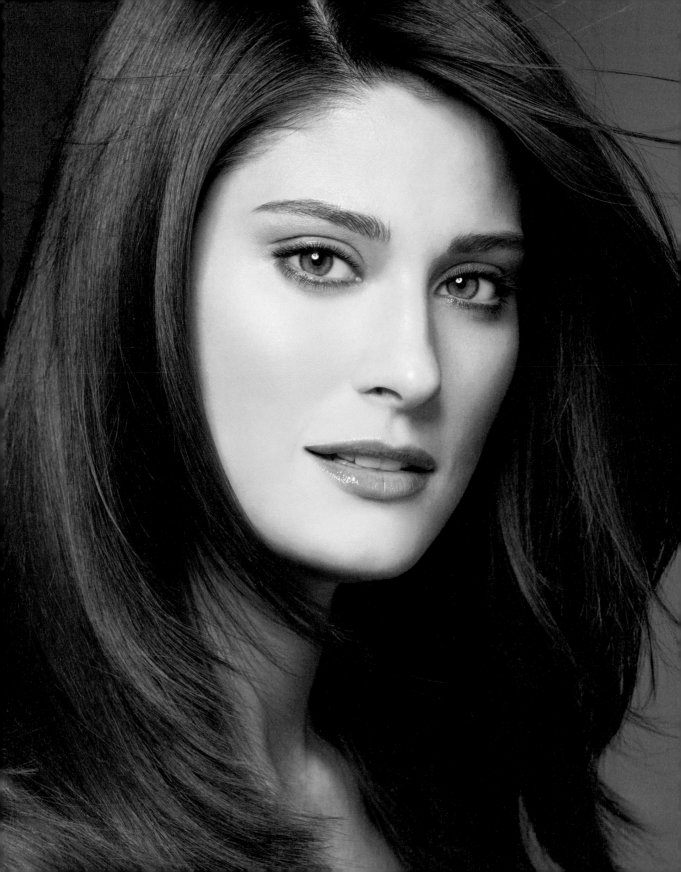

THIRTIES

Women in their thirties usually have the least amount of time to get ready in the morning. Raising young children, building a career, or both can sap every spare second. The 5-minute face is a savior for you and will keep you looking on top of your game.

Opposites Attract

With only five minutes to get ready you want to use less makeup with more impact. Use eye makeup colors that are the opposite of your natural eye hue. Smudge the shade into your lash line; your eyes will stand out with minimal effort. *If your eyes are blue*, choose chocolate brown; for *green eyes*, choose purples or plums; *hazel eyes* look amazing in greens; and *brown eyes* look beautiful in blues and forest greens. You'll be amazed by the payoff.

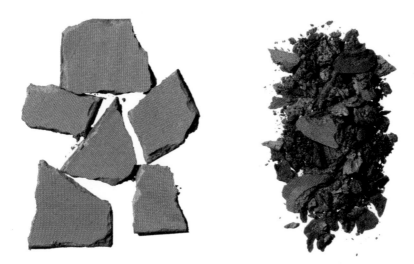

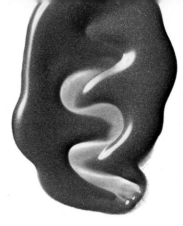

Glitter Be Gone

There is nothing worse than seeing a woman in her thirties wearing glitter. You can get away with it in your teens and twenties, but by thirty we should graduate to shimmer. Shimmer is more refined than chunky glitter and gives you a more polished and sophisticated glow. So when you're shopping for makeup, whether it's lip gloss or eye shadow, make sure the effect looks pearlescent on the skin, not like metallic confetti.

Day to Night

A lot of women in this age group find themselves going straight from the office to a night out on the town. Keep a small makeup bag in your desk drawer with a few extra products that will take your look up a notch (see the day-to-night look in chapter 7).

Sheer Radiance

Skin is less likely to have breakouts (except for the occasional monthly visitor) in this age group, so sheer tinted moisturizers are an ideal way to achieve a flawless complexion. Make sure to buy one with sunscreen.

FORTIES

Women in their forties know themselves well and usually feel the most confident with who they are. If not, then it's about time you do! Find your best feature and showcase it. If you don't know where to start, ask your friends' or family's opinion. Or think about what people have mentioned in the past. I bet you'll realize that you tend to receive compliments about a certain feature. Bingo!

Luminous Ladies

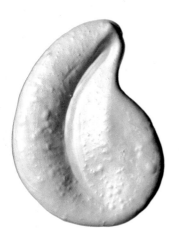

Skin's natural exfoliating process is slower now, and your complexion can look and feel dry. Besides stepping up your exfoliation routine (like adding glycolic peels into your skincare mix), start taking advantage of cream or liquid luminizers to add radiance. Apply luminizer to the tops of your cheekbones, but be careful not to cross over into the eye zone, where fine lines may show, since it may accentuate them. Then add a little luminizer under the arch of your eyebrow and on the inside corners of your eyes.

Moisture Whipped

Start choosing products that contain moisturizing and antiaging ingredients. Besides skincare there are plenty of foundations, concealers, and lip products out there that offer the deep hydration that your skin needs now to help soften lines, plump up sagginess, and reduce dullness. The more moisture you replace, the younger you will look.

> ### TIP
> Layering antiaging products can irritate some skins. If you notice redness or flakes, wear just one at a time.

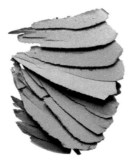

Get Cheeky

Bring back your youth and warm cheeks. Swirling on a soft blush to the apples of your cheeks is the best way to revive your complexion.

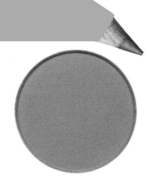

Wear Liner Longer

Is your eyeliner disappearing by the end of the day? Keep it in place by using a waterproof eyeliner pencil first. Then use an angle brush to sweep on the same color eye shadow over the liner for staying power. This will also keep the color true all day and night.

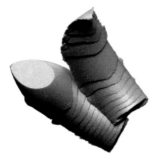

Lighten Up

Veer toward moisturizing lipstick formulas in lighter, more natural shades. Choose ones that offer a pearly finish; they look soft and sophisticated. Avoid dark matte lips, which can be aging, and wet-finish glosses, which look inappropriate now as we mature.

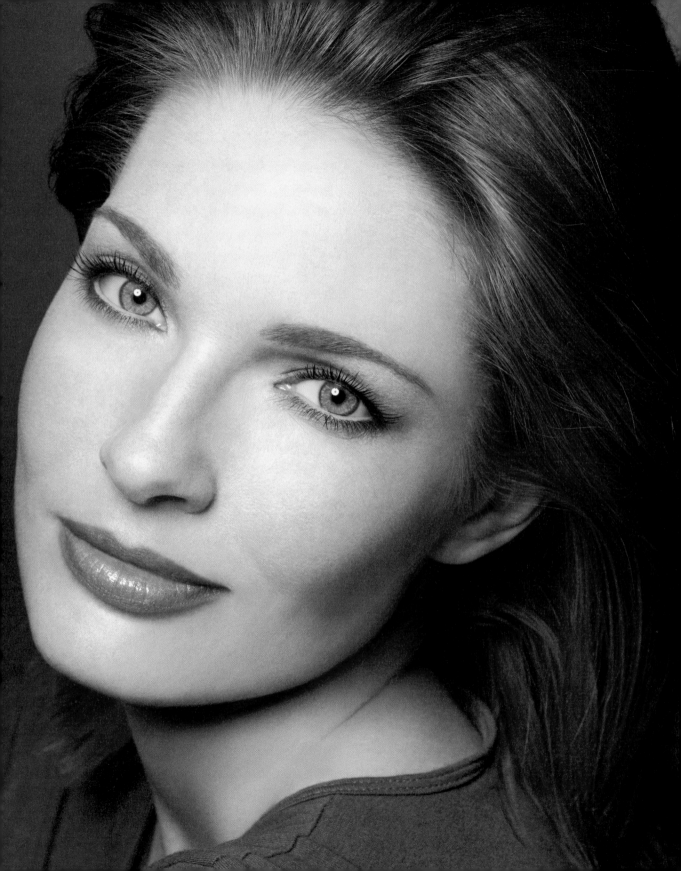

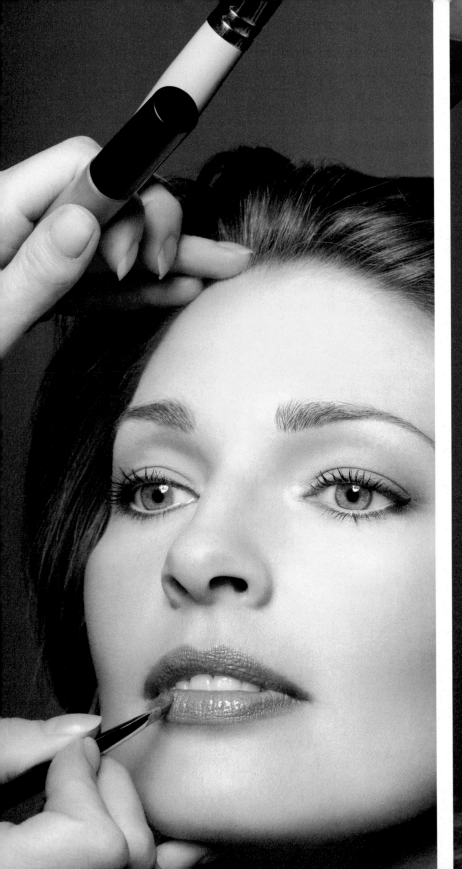
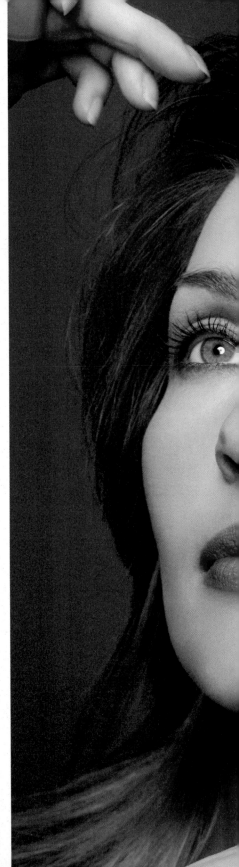

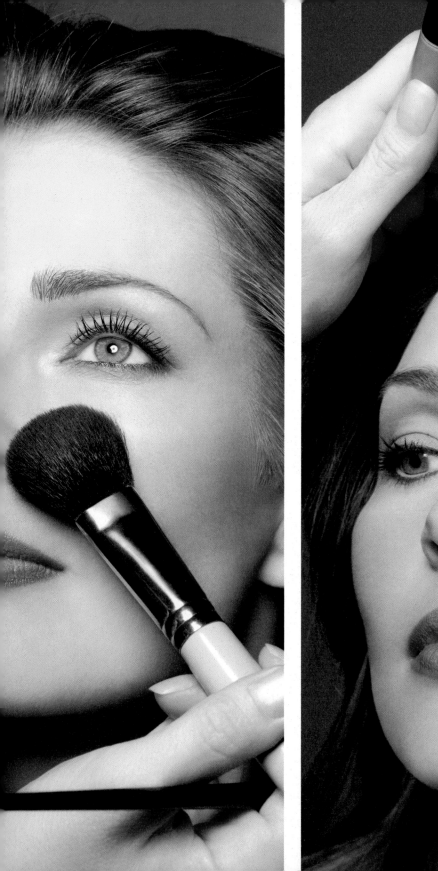
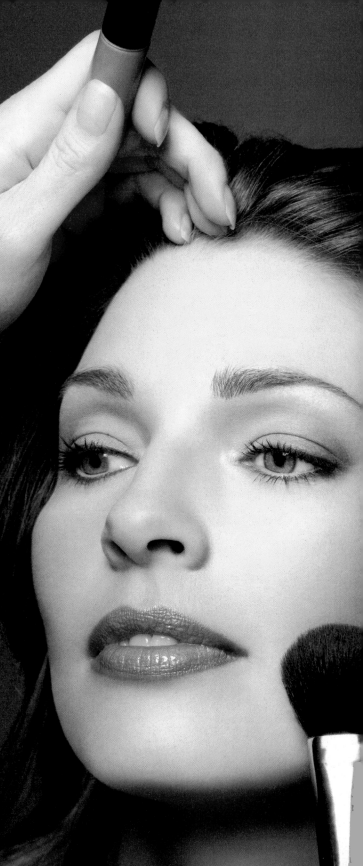

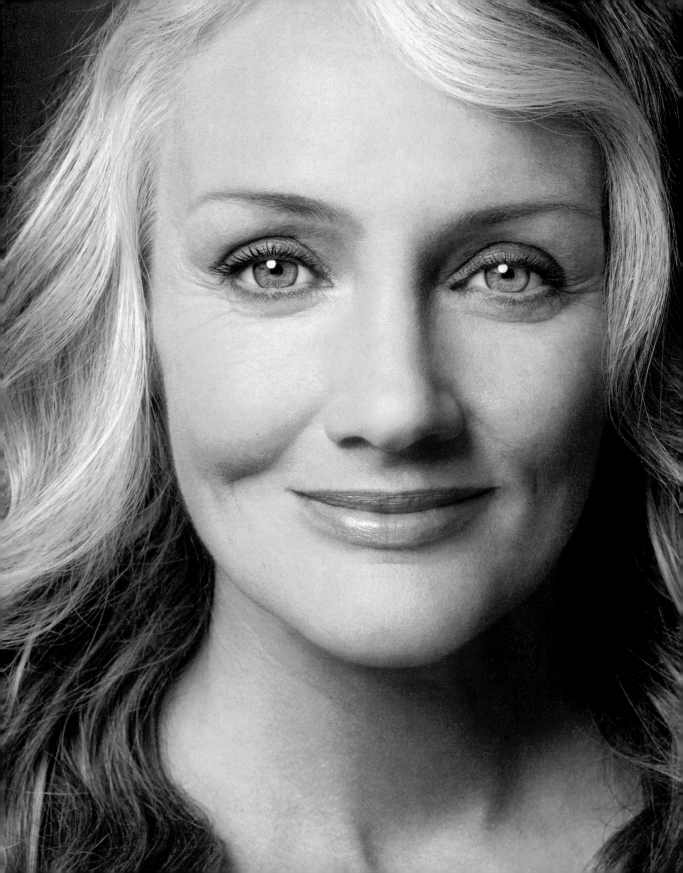

FIFTIES

In your fifties, the secret to beauty is living a healthy lifestyle and letting the joy show on your face. Confidence, a great smile, and laugh lines (which you've *earned*) will keep you looking gorgeous no matter what gravity has in store for you. As we mature, our skin loses a bit of its natural color. Luckily, restoring radiance is not hard at all.

The Right Blush and Lip Color: Think Rosy

Rose-colored blush and lips make skin look it's best—they instantly brighten your whole face. Choose *cream* formula blush over powder; the dewier texture will look softer on your skin. Also, pick moisturizing lipsticks, which will look beautiful and sophisticated, to boot. Pass on high shine lip glosses, which can look a bit vampy.

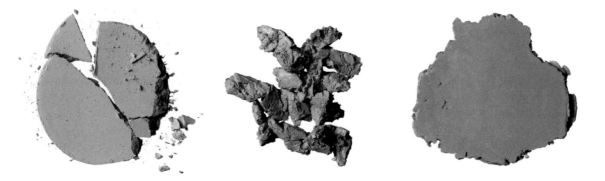

Sneaky Lip-Liner Trick

To prevent lipstick from bleeding, trace your natural lip line with a lip-colored pencil, then add lipstick. The waxiness of the pencil will seal the lipstick in place, and unlike colored liners, a lip-colored pencil won't leave you with "ring around the mouth" if your lipstick wears off during the day.

Say No to Tattooed-on Makeup

Never opt for permanent makeup! As we age our skin loses elasticity and droops a bit, so permanent eyebrows could wind up lower than they were originally.

Vanishing Brows

Brows can become sparse with time, and their natural color may fade slightly. To bring back definition, skip brow powder and instead use longer-lasting waterproof liquid brow corrector or a brow pencil. If your hair is gray, choose a taupe or blonde shade to fill brows in for a natural look. Check out chapter 2 for more brow tips.

Brighten Your Smile

You can take ten years off your look by whitening your teeth. It will erase the yellowish cast from coffee, tea, cola, red wine, and cigarettes. Consider a service from your dentist (like laser whitening or bleaching trays) or try whitening strips that you can use at home. These products are a cheaper option than going to the dentist and work amazingly well.

Mascara Meltdown

To prevent mascara from smudging, wear a waterproof formula on your upper lash line only. It will resist smears better. Leave your lower lashes bare; instead smudge waterproof pencil along the lower lashline for definition. It won't budge.

A Word About Anything Sparkly

Makeup with loads of shimmer won't flatter you now. The glittery particles tend to settle into lines, making them more noticeable. A better option is to use light-reflective makeup (like foundation), which is described in the Secret Weapon section of chapter 3. Follow the highlighter steps in chapter 4 to create a luminous effect.

Fast Fix

FIVE-SECOND FACE-LIFT: Right after foundation, apply a light concealer pencil along the creases that run from the side of your nose down to the corner of your mouth (called the nasal labial folds). Do the same from the outer corner of each eye up to the end of your brows. Blend with your finger so the highlighter looks like part of your own skin. The result? This will lift the outer corners of the eyes and bounce light off the folds around the mouth, making it look like you have had "work" done without the work.

Magnify

A small magnifying mirror can make a huge difference in your blending results, especially for women who wear glasses. Try one, and you'll see how much easier it is to stroke on mascara and smudge and soften eyeliner, brow colors, and highlighter.

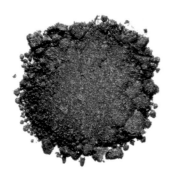
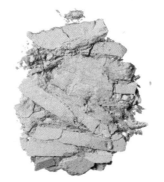

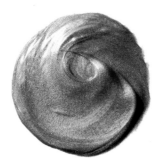
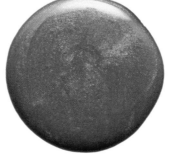
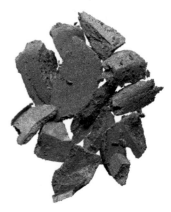
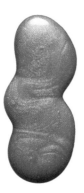
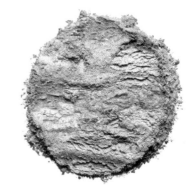
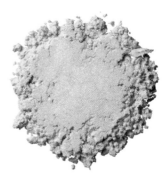
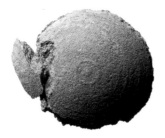
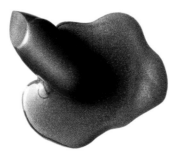

chapter seven

SPECIAL OCCASION LOOKS

Once you've mastered the 5-minute face, check out these other looks. Each one starts with the 5-minute face—you just add an extra minute here and there. You won't believe how fast and easy it is to create so many different looks!

CLASSIC BLACK-TIE PARTY

They don't happen every day, but when black-tie events do come up, we want to look amazing. Think old-time Hollywood glamour! It's all about the red lips and false lashes for this look—easier than you think, I promise. Every woman can pull this off—you'll have people raving from the moment you walk in.

Get the Look

- Start with the first five steps of the 5-minute face: foundation, under-eye concealer, spot concealer, powder, and highlighter.

- Cut a set of false lashes in half, and use only the half with the *shorter* lashes. Apply a small bit of lash adhesive along the upper strip. You'll find natural-looking lash strips at drugstores; adhesive is usually included.

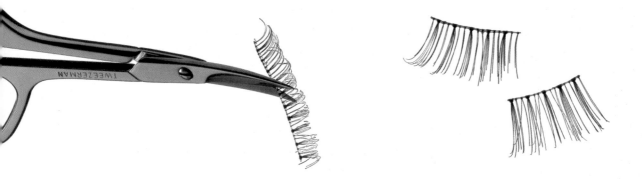

- Look down, and gently press the upper strip along the outer half of your own upper lashes—the fakes should lay against your lash roots, with no gap. After the glue has dried, sweep black cream eyeliner (it is easier and more natural looking than liquid) along the upper lash line to hide the seam where the false lashes and the roots meet.

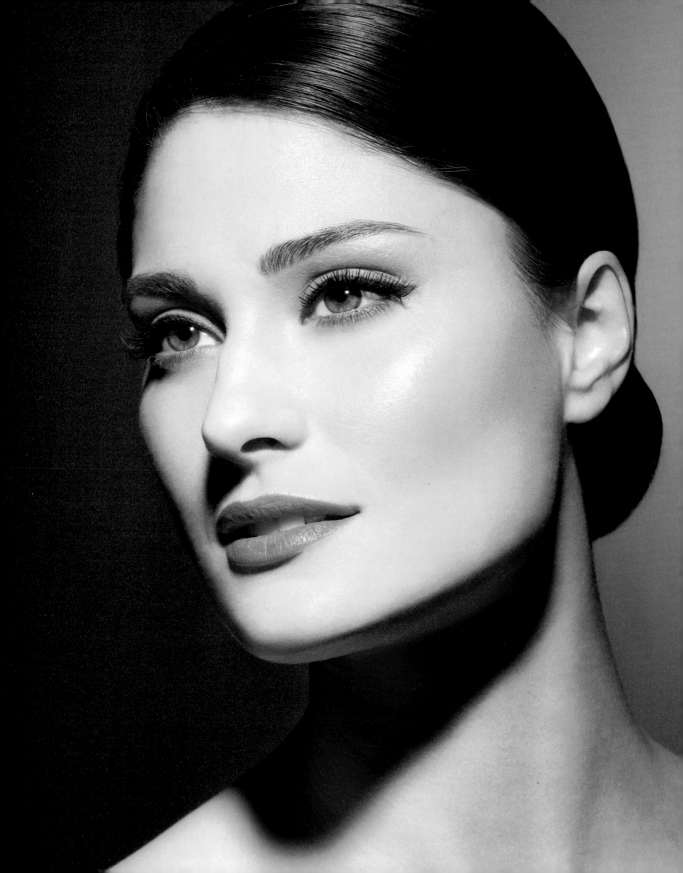

- Smudge light brown eye shadow across your eyelid and under your lower lashes.

- Sweep on a coat of black mascara to blend the fakes with your real ones. Don't use mascara on the lower lashes; your eyes will look overdone.

- Apply red lipstick. Use a small lip brush for a perfect finish.

- Now for blush. I like to save this step for last. The reason? Red lipstick adds a lot of color to your face and you may not need as much blush as you'd think. I like to go more subtle than usual with a peach tone, so the focus stays on the lips and eyes.

TIP

Bring a piece of white paper to the store and swipe testers on it. When viewing the red against white, it will be easier to detect if there is a blue (cool) or yellow (warm) tint in the product.

THE RIGHT RED

All women can wear red lipstick no matter what shape their lips are or what coloring they have. For red-shy women, try one that's super sheer, like a sheer lipstick or a stain. For all-out glamour, choose a classic, cream-finish lipstick. For help choosing the right shade of red:

Fair complexions are flattered by *cool reds* (like cherry or the color of a red rose)

Redheads look great wearing *warm* reds (like tomato or brick)

Medium or olive skin looks best with *classic true reds* (like an apple)

Dark skin can pull off *deep reds* with ease

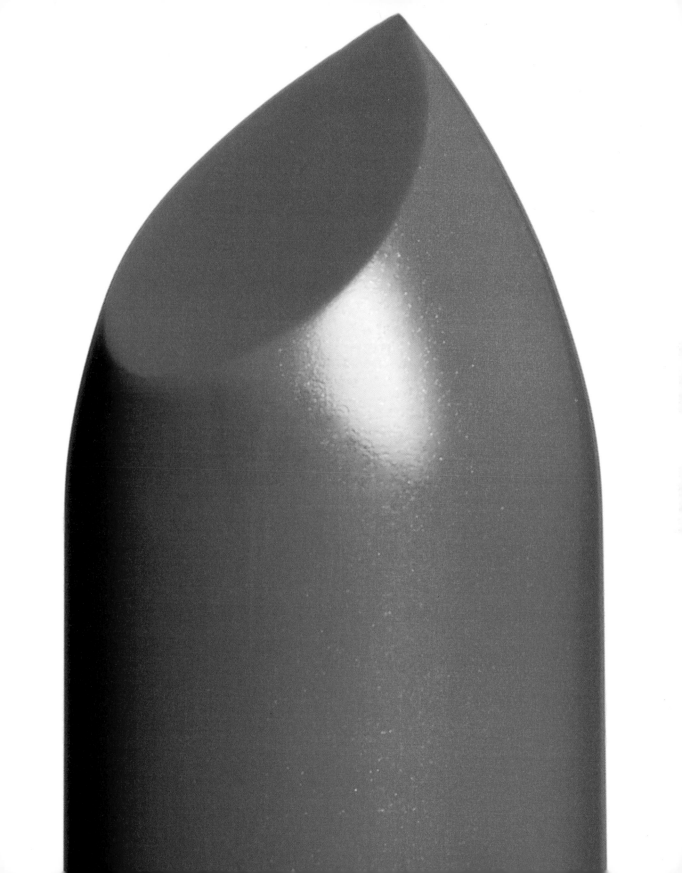

Black-tie Nails

Match your nails to your red lip shade—it's a classic look. Just keep nails on the short side. Long red talons look too Elvira-ish. Another color option for fingers or toes: sheer nude polish, which won't compete with your lips.

MAKE RED LIP COLOR LAST LONGER

Nothing draws attention to your mouth like red lips. Make sure your lips are smooth to begin with, and, since the bold color will show any mistakes, apply red lip color very precisely. You'll do just fine with a small brush, as I've instructed, but if you want the *ultimate* application, here's how you can go to town in five steps:

1. Buff bare lips with a Q-tip dipped into a little petroleum jelly and sugar.

2. Apply red lip stain. Lip stains are usually liquid or gels that stain the lips red, creating a waterproof smudgeproof finish. It will act like a backup in case your lip color wears off.

3. Lightly line lips with a soft red lip liner—follow your natural outline. It will act like a gate to keep color from seeping out, then fill in the lips with the liner. Blot with a makeup sponge to make sure you have a soft-looking base. It should not look harshly drawn on.

4. Apply red lipstick with a lip brush. It will offer precise results. I prefer moisturizing cream lipstick. A glossy finish with red lips can look too gaudy.

5. If you stray out of line (red can stain skin), "clean up" around your mouth with a little foundation. Apply it with a thin concealer brush.

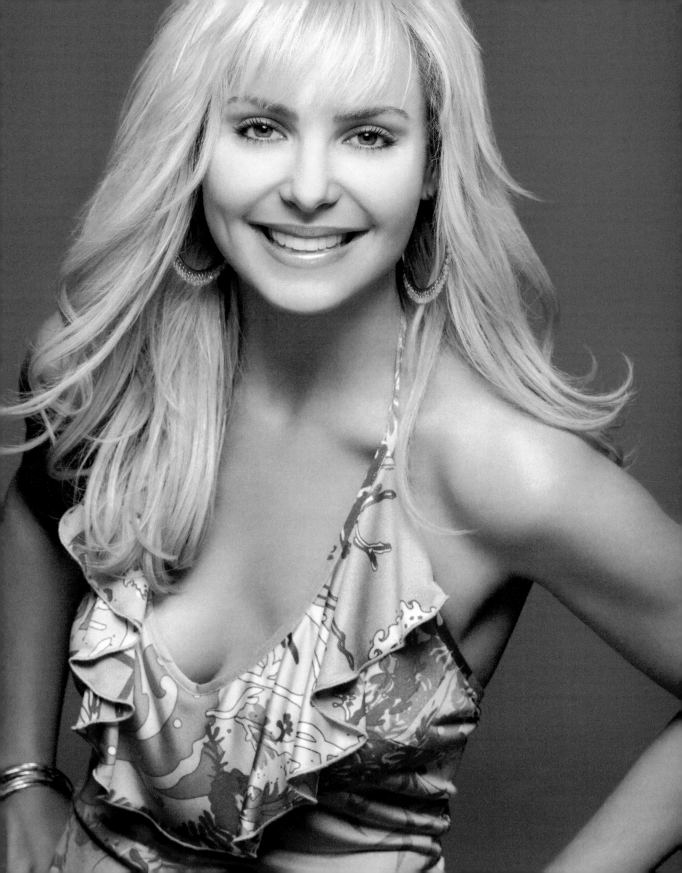

VACATION GLOW

Some women believe that taking bronzer on vacation is like taking sand to the beach. Well, whether you're on a tropical island or bopping around your hometown in the summer heat, you should *always* fake your tan! Remember, there is no beauty in skin cancer, so please keep yourself protected with high SPF sunscreen and take advantage of the natural, healthy results that self-tanners and bronzers offer. Here's the best way to fake it.

Get the Look

- Apply self-tanner (see chapter 1 for application techniques) the night before leaving for your beachy paradise (or barbecue). By the time you wake up, you'll have a golden tan.

- Follow the first four steps of the 5-minute face, but instead of using foundation, try a tinted moisturizer with SPF (that matches your faux-tanned skin) to give you a more natural look. Use your under-eye concealer and spot concealer, then powder lightly in the areas where you tend to get the most shiny. *Skip highlighter.* Your skin will take on a glow of it's own in hot weather.

- Sweep on powder bronzer with a big fluffy powder brush along your temples, under your cheekbones, and lightly across your forehead, nose, and chin. Go easy so you won't look too dark.

- Next, apply pink powder blush to the apples of your cheeks.

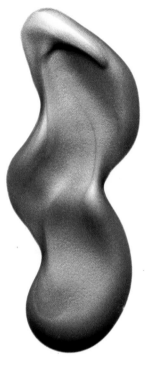

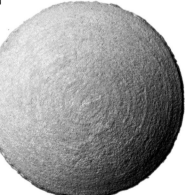

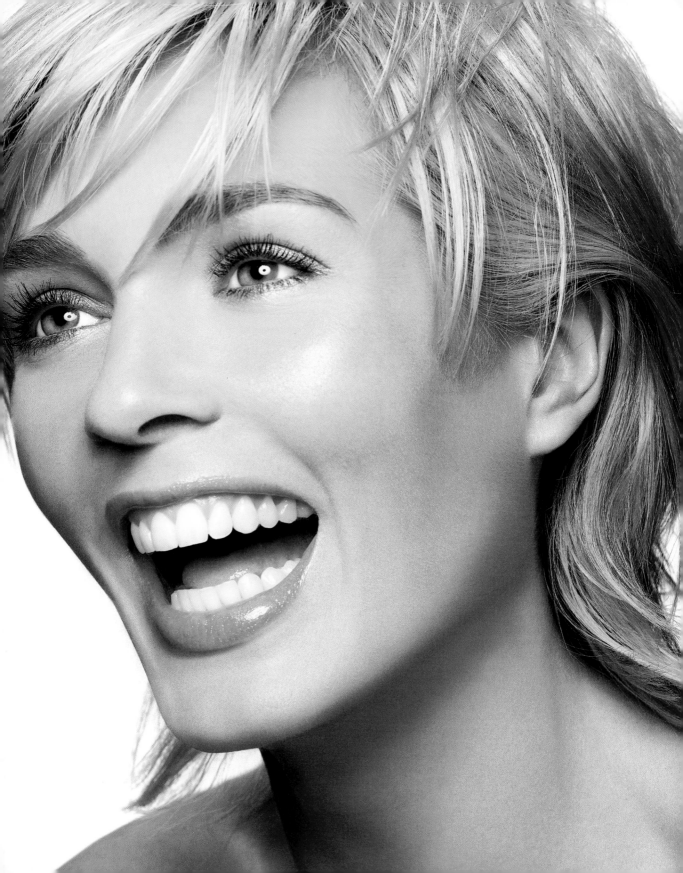

PEDICURE POINTERS

Pretty seashell, coral, or pink nail polish will look beautiful with a tan.

THROW OIL-BLOTTING PAPERS INTO YOUR BAG

They act like a sponge and lift away greasiness, so you don't have to apply powder all day. Powder will begin to look cakey and heavy if you load it on.

- Dust a light sweep of gold eye shadow across your lids, and skip eyeliner.

- Apply waterproof mascara to your top lashes only.

- For lips, use sheer berry lip gloss or tinted balm. Either way, choose one with an SPF.

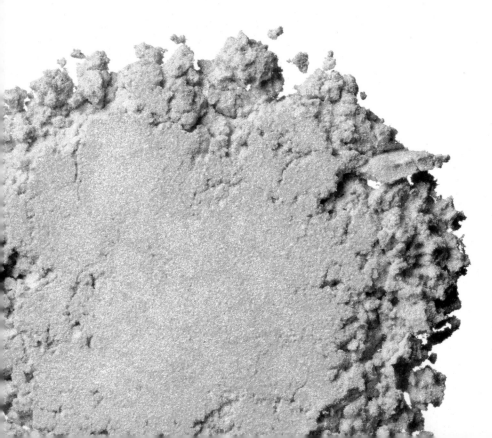

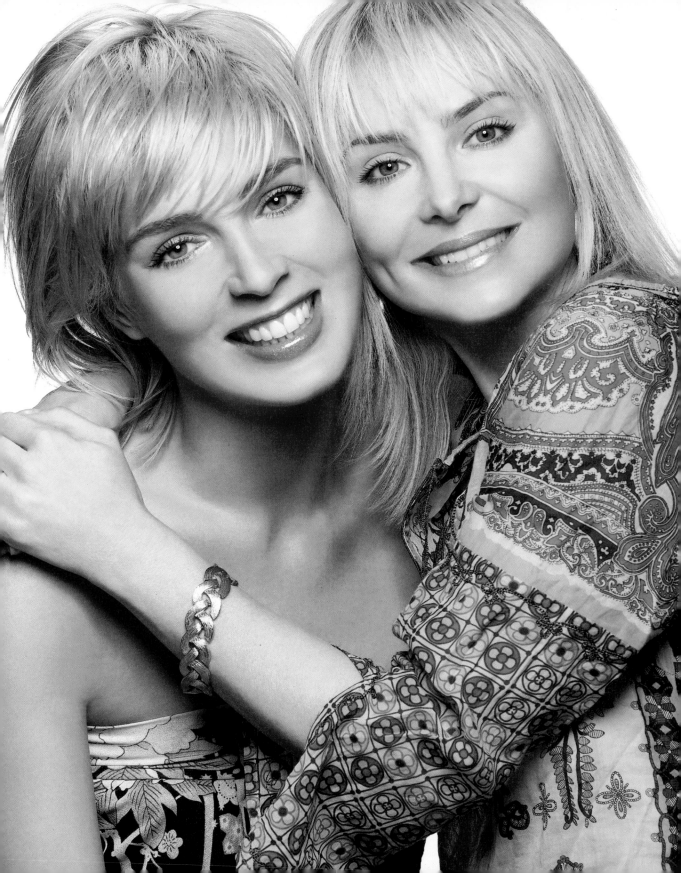

WEDDING

This is your special day, and you want to look the best you ever have! There's no need to spend a ton of extra money on a professional makeup artist. You can do it yourself: all you need are a few makeup tricks that will get you glowing for those picture-perfect moments, and will help you look amazing in photos.

Get the Look

- Apply shimmering body lotion from your neck down as soon as you hop out of the shower. Your skin will look soft and gleamy all day and night.

- Follow the first five steps of the 5-minute face: foundation, under-eye concealer, spot concealer, powder, and highlighter.

- Next, sweep a tawny pink eye shadow across your eyelids from the lash line to the crease.

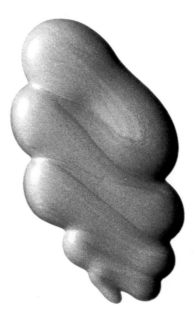

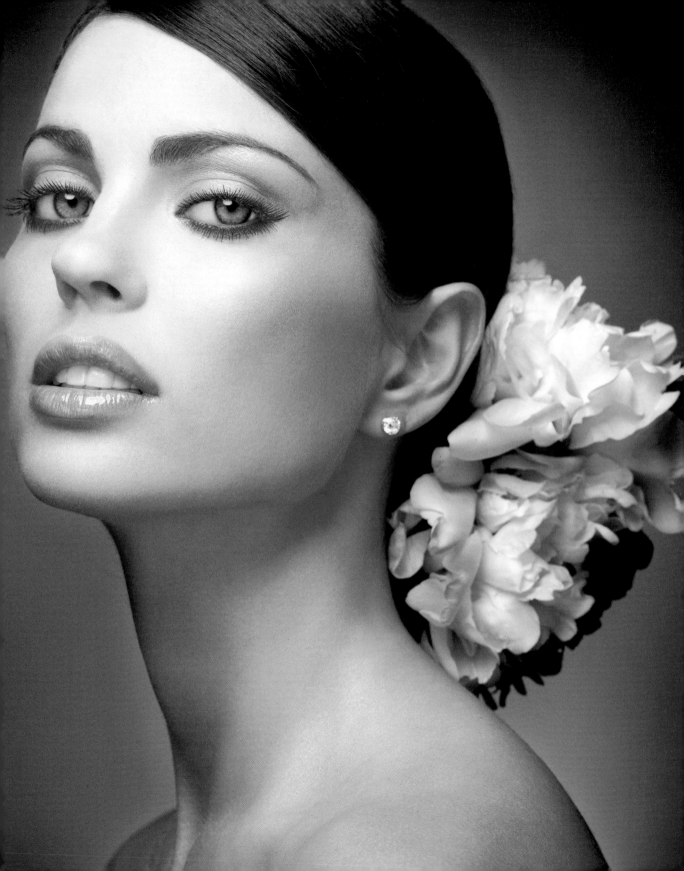

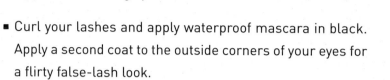

- Apply a burgundy-brown waterproof eyeliner pencil along your upper lash line, and wing it out a bit at the ends. Then trace over the eye liner using an angled brush dipped in matching eye shadow color to soften the line.

- Curl your lashes and apply waterproof mascara in black. Apply a second coat to the outside corners of your eyes for a flirty false-lash look.

- Dust rose-colored powder blush on the apples of your cheeks and along your cheekbones. You'll want it to look a little bit more intense than usual, but don't go crazy. (Practice your makeup ahead of time—have a friend snap some photos so you can see how much blush you need to apply.)

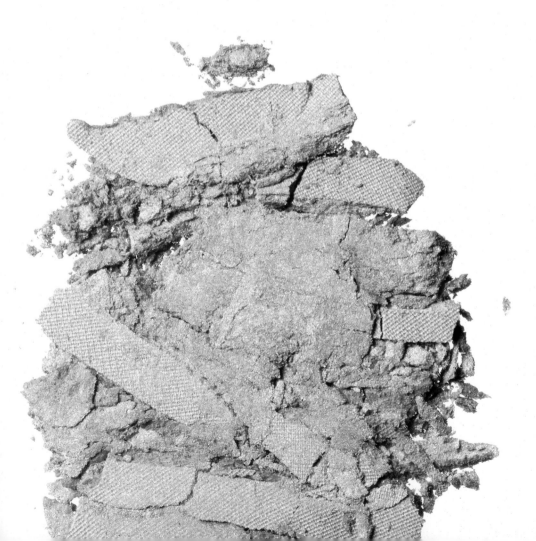

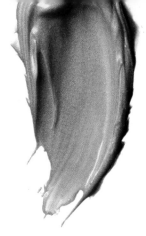

- Outline, then fill in your lips with a natural, lip-colored lip liner, which will provide a base for your lipstick so it stays on longer. Next, sweep on a soft, shimmering pink-rose colored lipstick, and add a small dab of shimmering gloss to the center of your lower lip. Now, with a very thin brush or Q-tip, add a dab of the same highlighter used in the 5-minute face on the top of the Cupid's bow of your upper lip (the top of the "V") and at the center under the lower lip. This will capture light, giving the illusion of full, pouty lips.

- Ask one of your bridesmaids to carry your lipstick, gloss, powder, and a few Q-tips for touch-ups throughout the night.

WEDDING DAY DISASTERS . . . AVOIDED!

Try these beauty helpers a solid month beforehand. This way, if there are any glitches, you'll have plenty of time to work out the kinks.

1. **Self-tanner:** whether you use a bottle or visit a spray-on booth, you'll want to make sure the color is natural.

2. **Deep exfoliation, like glycolic peels:** although these treatments are gentle, you never know how your skin will react. You don't want any irritation or flakes (old, dull skin sheds for a day or two after each treatment) to show on your special day. Four weeks gives you time for a few prewedding treatments.

3. **Facials:** I find that facials can cause skin to break out, since some skin types overreact to the extreme cleaning.

4. **Waxing:** to avoid rashes and red welts, make sure all hair removal is done well ahead of time.

BIG DAY NO-NO'S

- Say no to cream eye shadow or blush for today—they don't have the intensity that powders do.

- Avoid super glossy or super dark lips. They're too high maintenance. You have to remember, you'll be kissing your new husband, friends, and family, and you'll be sipping toast after toast.

- Another reason to choose lighter over dark hues: lighter shades don't require the same upkeep as darker ones do. You won't notice if your pink lipstick has faded a tad, the way you would red.

- Stay away from false lashes. You may cry (you'll never know until you're standing by your groom's side), and tears can make false lashes crawl down your cheeks.

- There's a difference between glitter (chunky, obviously shiny flecks) and shimmer (powdery-fine shine that's subtle and luminous). Choose shimmer. This is your wedding, not a New Year's Eve blast.

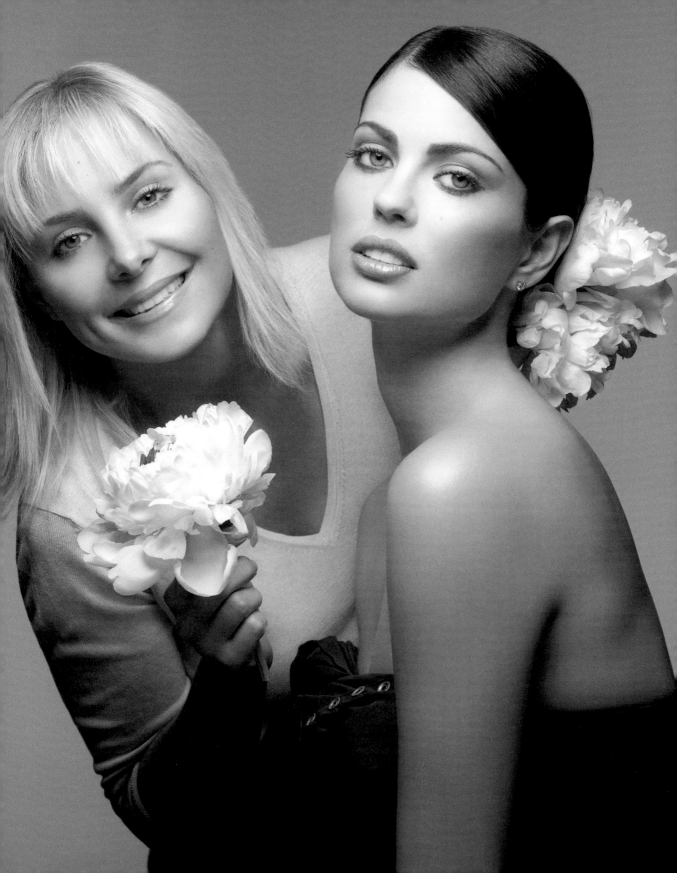

TAKE YOUR LOOK FROM DAY TO NIGHT

There are times when you have to leave straight from work to attend a dinner, a party, or even your kid's school play. By adding a few quick steps to the 5-minute face you applied in the morning, you can transform yourself from day to night in no time at all.

Get the Look

- Use oil-blotting papers to soak up any greasy areas. Next, use a concealer brush dipped in a little foundation to smooth out any makeup that may have seeped into fine lines or under your eyes. Touch up areas of redness or dark circles the same way.

- Add evening drama to your eyes with dark eyeliner (like black or eggplant). Sweep it along your lash line, on top of your day liner. *If you have almond shaped or round eyes*, add a smoky effect by lining your eyes' inner rims. *If your eyes are smaller,* just line the upper lash line and wing it out a bit at the ends. Next, apply a shimmering eye shadow in an evening shade, like a sparkling smoky taupe, from your upper lash line up to the crease, and under your lower lash line.

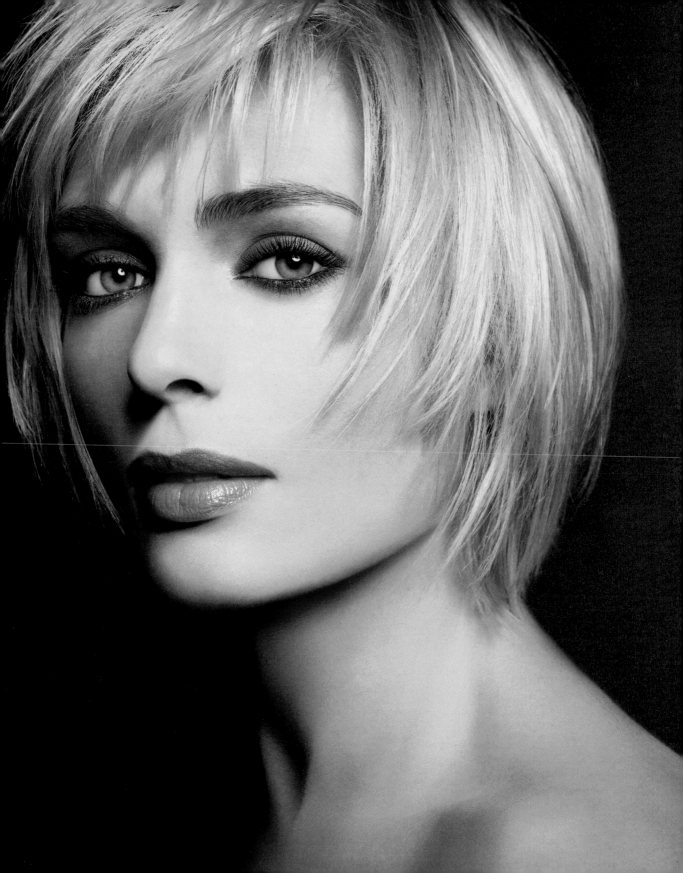

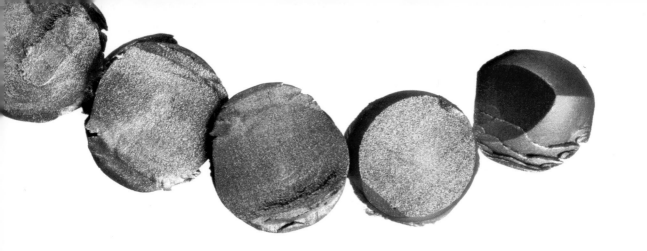

- Sweep a bit more highlight powder on top of your cheekbones, under your eyebrows, and by your tear ducts, just like you did in the morning. (I prefer powder over cream for an evening look because the color pigments in powder are more intense.) Dust the highlight powder onto your décolletage area for a sexy glow.

- Swirl on a bit more blush.

- Apply a slightly deeper shade of lipstick or choose a lip gloss to add a sexy touch.

- Add a light dusting of translucent powder to your T-zone and a spritz of your favorite scent, and you're gorgeously good to go!

WHAT *NOT* TO ADD AT YOUR DESK

There is no need to reapply mascara—it will just look clumpy. Let the dark eyeliner add the "pop." Foundation will still look fresh just by spot-concealing; evening light is more forgiving than daylight.

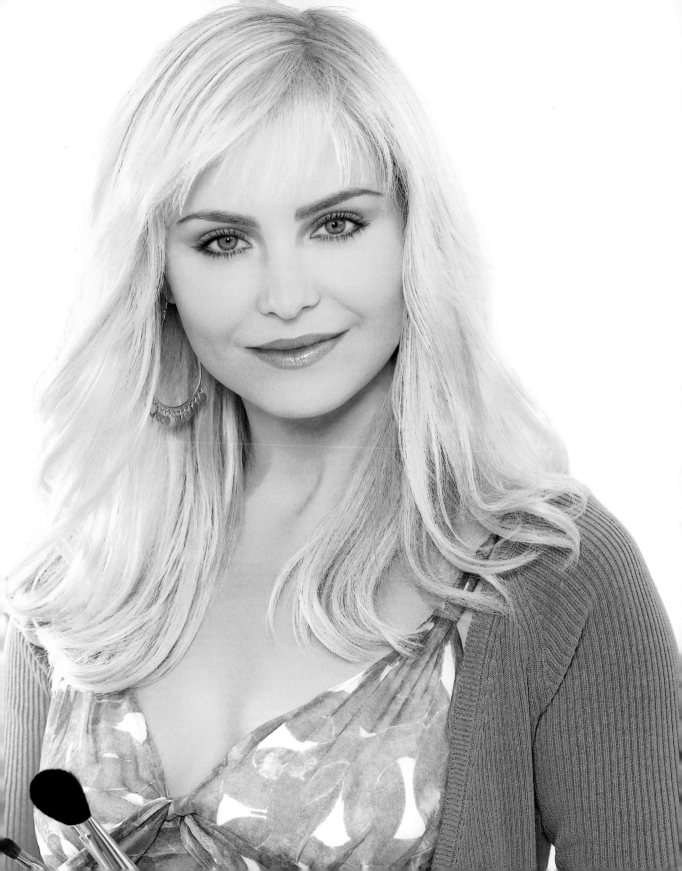

HOLIDAY FACE

Holidays are the best time to experiment and play with looks you may have been afraid to try in the past. Because it's a festive occasion, you can get away with almost anything in the name of fun. For example, I love this look—it has an alluring 1920s feel, with a light, modern twist.

Get the Look

- Follow all the steps in the 5-minute face: foundation, under-eye concealer, spot concealer, powder, highlighter, blush, eyeliner, mascara, and lip color. *Don't apply mascara until the end.*

- Now, sweep on a shade of plum eye shadow from your upper lash line to your crease and smudge under the lower lash line.

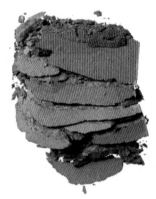

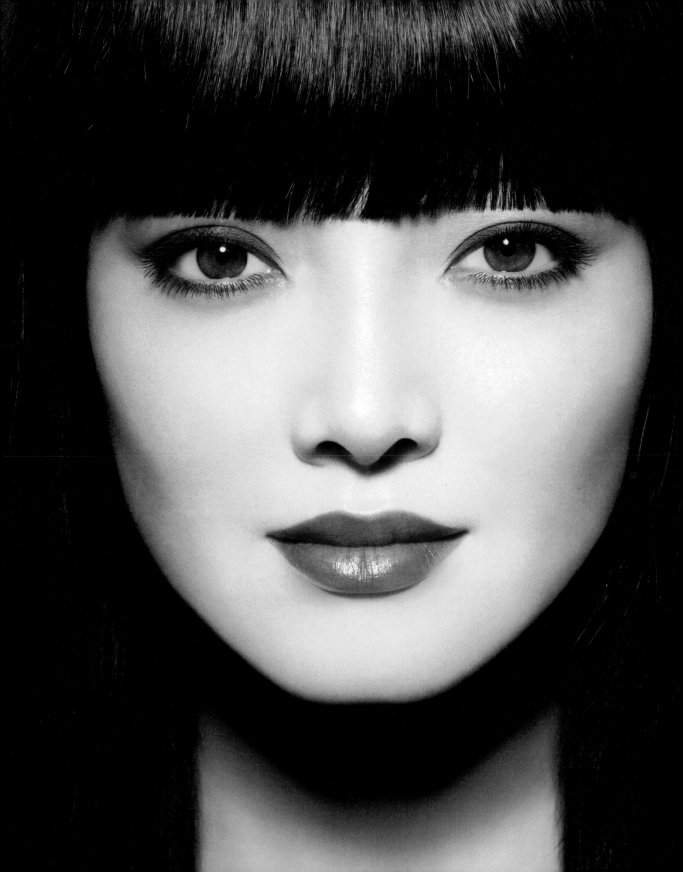

- Apply a deep plum lip stain to your lips, but skip gloss because it would be overkill.

- Apply two coats of black mascara.

How to Make It All Work Together

If you choose a daring makeup look, let your face be the star of the show and go simple with your hair; try a style that's sleek and understated, like a pretty, low chignon. Jewelry should follow suit.

SOME HOLIDAY-FUN LOOKS TO PLAY AROUND WITH

Dark lips	Retro looks	Liquid eyeliner
False lashes	Sparkling lip glosses	Dark nail polish
Smoky eye shadow	Body shimmer	

chapter eight

TRENDS THAT WORK

Along with the latest fashion styles, makeup trends create a buzz every spring and fall. *"It's all about a smoky eye,"* or *"Tangerine is so right now"* but how does the hoopla translate in real life? Just because some model went traipsing down a runway wearing bright orange lipstick, should you be wearing it, too? The key to interpreting the trends is to learn how to turn them from runway to real life. The looks here are "trends" that have (and will continue to) withstand the test of time—there's something here for everyone. Enjoy!

SMOKY EYES

At some point we all want to try the smoky eye. It's sexy, smoldery—what's not to like? But go too heavy with the dark hues and you can wind up looking like you've been in a bar brawl. *Not* a good look. Women with closely set or very small eyes ought to avoid this option altogether because it can look too overwhelming. (Don't worry, there are other trends for you to play with!) For the rest of you, here are the basic steps for creating the smoky eye.

Get the Look

- Start with the first five steps of the 5-minute face: foundation, under-eye concealer, spot concealer, powder, and highlighter.

- Next, line your upper and lower lash line (right into the roots of the lashes) with dark eyeliner, such as black or chocolate brown. Smudge it with an angled brush (or a Q-tip), so the line is soft.

- If you have large eyes, line the inner rim with black eyeliner for an extra sultry look.

- Apply matching dark eye shadow from your lash line up to the crease, and sweep under the lower lashline to soften the pencil.

- Now use a softer color in the same family, such as burgundy brown or eggplant, and sweep it into the crease.

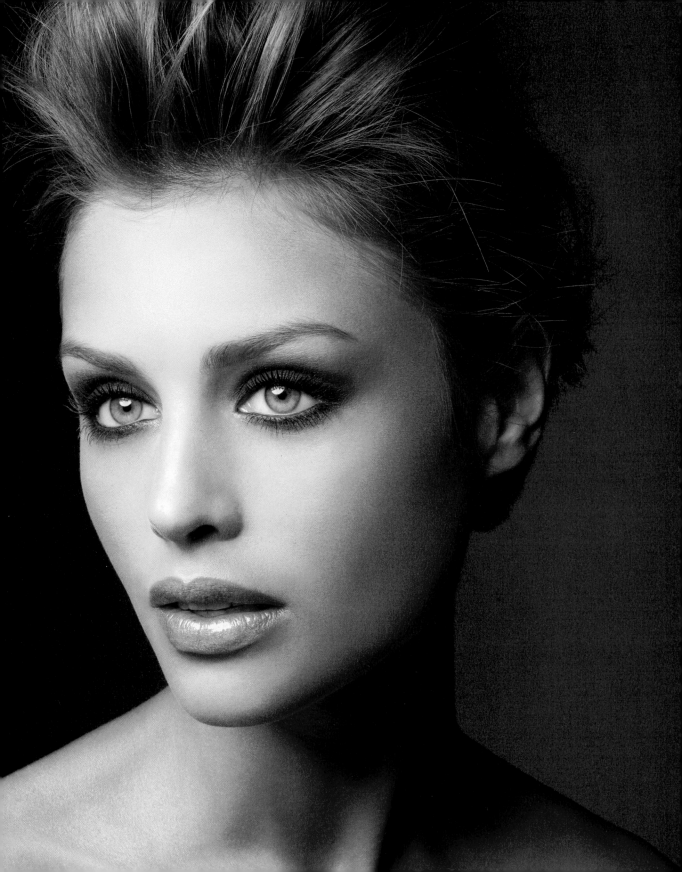

- Add another sweep of shimmery highlighter under the arch of each brow and to your eyes' inner corners, by the tear ducts.

- Blend, blend, blend together so there is a gradation of color, from darkest at the lash line to lightest under brow.

- Sweep black mascara on the top and bottom lashes.

- Last, swipe on a pearly sheer plum lip gloss.

Fast Fix

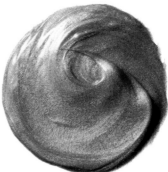

MAGIC ERASER: Use a sponge dipped into a little foundation and under-eye concealer to clean up any shadow that has fallen under your eyes during application for a flawless, clean finish.

SMOKY EYES COLOR TIP

You don't have to wear black, charcoal, or brown eye shadow to achieve a smoky look; all kinds of hues, from plums to greens to blues, will work. The key is to keep the liners and the shadows in the same color family. See chapter 5 to learn the best colors for your eyes.

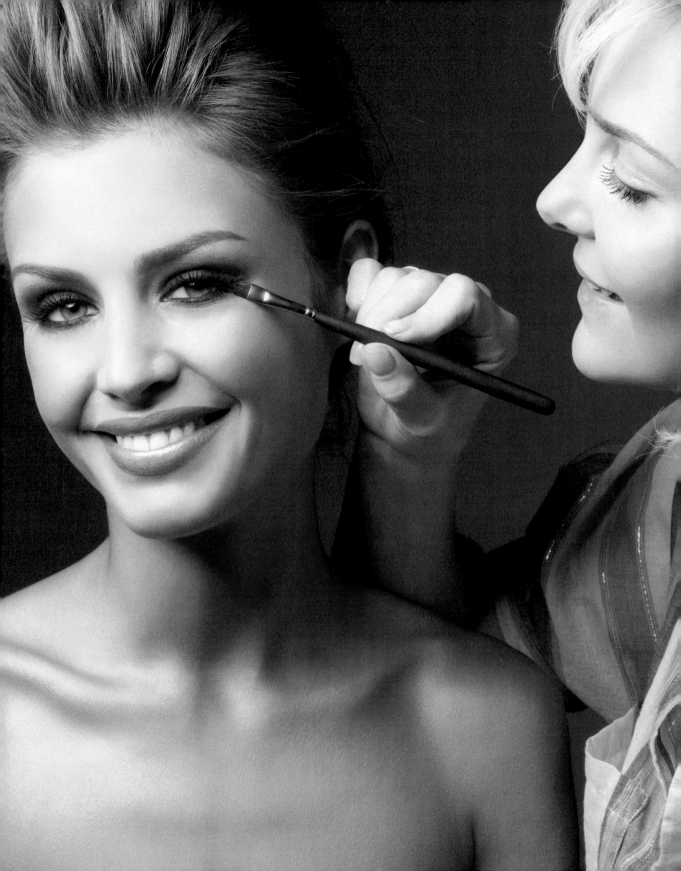

NUDES

Nude makeup made its big debut in the early nineties and was a success because it was a way for a woman to appear like she was naturally flawless and not wearing any makeup at all. The only problem was that back then, colors tended to look matted and chalky and made everyone appear a little pasty. Makeup technology has advanced, and the "new" nudes are ultra sheer with light-reflecting pigments that add radiance for a more polished finish. Tip: choose nude shades that have a hint of peach or pink so they will enhance your skin and won't wash you out.

Get the Look

Follow the first five steps of the 5-minute face: foundation, under-eye concealer, spot concealer, powder, and highlighter.

- Next, sweep a soft, shimmering, toffee-colored eye shadow from lash line to crease.

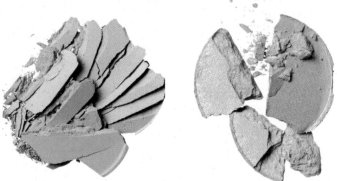

- Smudge dark chocolate pencil into your lash line. Eyeliner is key with bare makeup, so your eyes don't disappear.

- Sweep black mascara on upper *and* lower lashes.

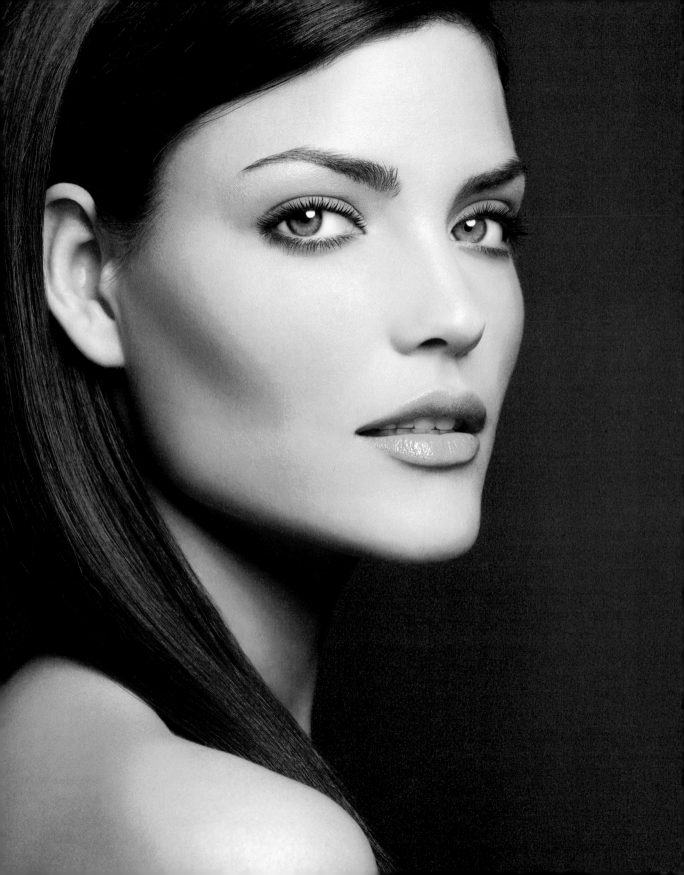

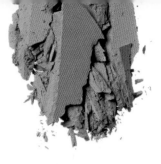

- Apply soft, sandy pink blush onto the apples of your cheeks and slightly upward along your cheekbones. It will give your face an extra hint of color so you don't look pale.

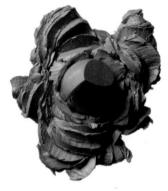

- Last, choose a sheer nude moisturizing lip color. A gleamy finish is essential with nude shades because it will help your lips stand out.

Best Nude Lip Colors

Porcelain-skinned redheads, blondes, and fair-skinned brunettes look lovely with *peachy nudes*.
Brunettes with olive skin look beautiful with *warm pink nudes*.
Dark-skinned women look amazing wearing *mocha tones*.

Feature Focus

The nude look shown here is very subtle but can be intensified by choosing one feature to enhance more than the others. For instance, if your cheekbones are amazing, swirl a little more blush onto the apples of your cheeks to make them the focal point. If it's your lips, add a sheer nude gloss for extra sexiness. Because of the monochromatic appearance of this trend, it will never look like you have gone overboard.

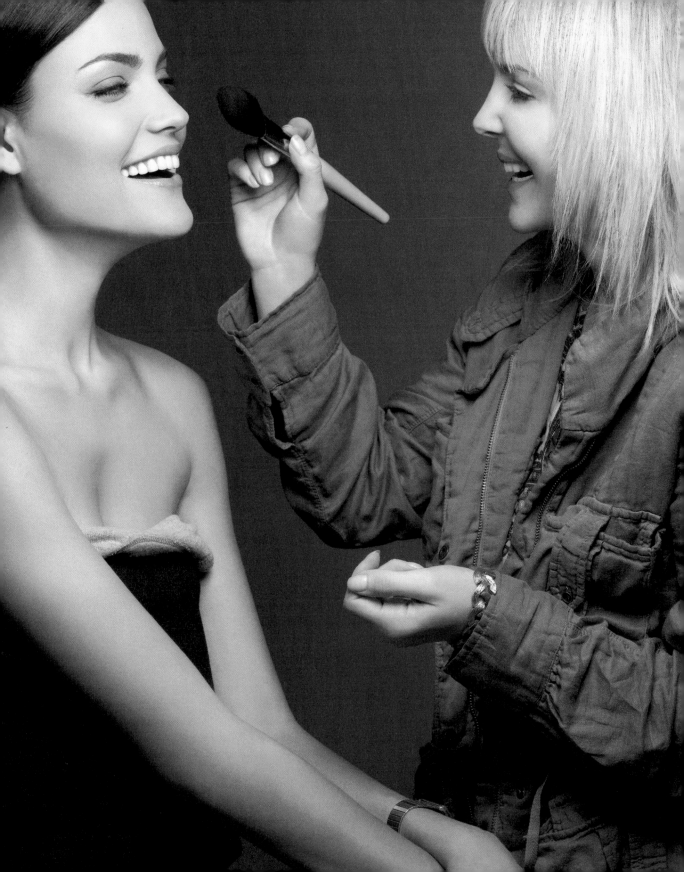

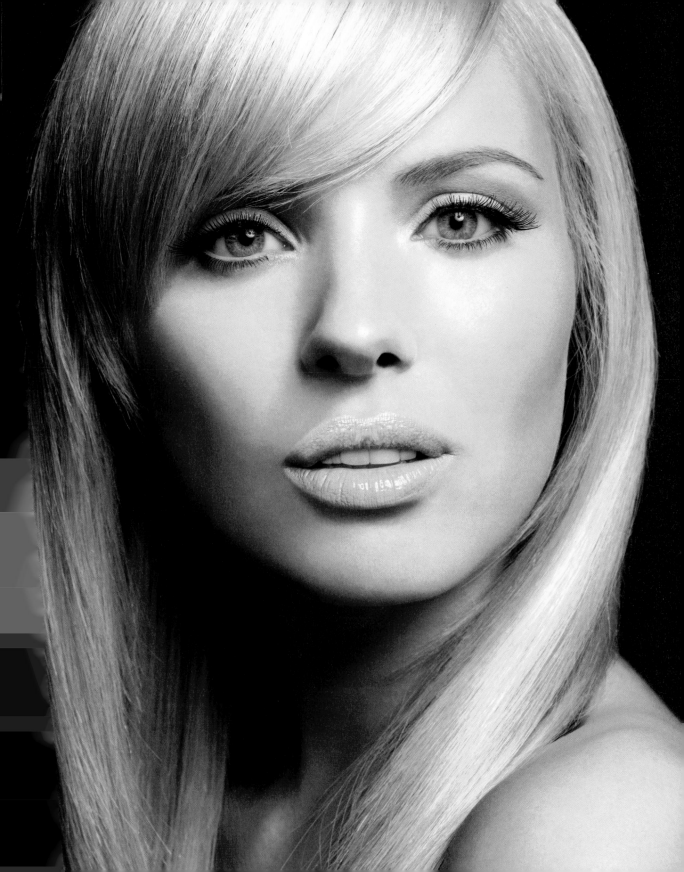

RETRO SIXTIES

Retro trends come and go, but there is always something classically sexy about them. Channeling your inner Brigitte Bardot can do a lot for your self-esteem, and hey—it's fun to look a little different from time to time! The retro sixties look still works today, but what makes it modern here is the combination of sheer makeup textures and a lighter application technique, which will look more natural and fresh than the opaque and heavy look offered in the original era.

Get the Look

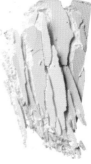

Follow the first five steps of the the 5-minute face: foundation, under-eye concealer, spot concealer, powder, and highlighter.

- Sweep a sheer matte vanilla eye shadow from your lash line to the crease.

- Add taupe eye shadow to the crease.

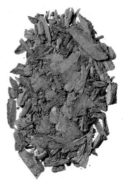

- Apply false lashes to the outer half of your upper lash line. See the false lash tips for the classic black-tie look detailed in chapter 7.

- Hide the seam where the false lashes sit on your own lashes with a little black liquid eyeliner.

- Brush on two to three coats of black mascara to your upper and lower lashes. Wait a few seconds in between coats so the mascara has a chance to dry just a bit. This will give you that spiky sixties lash look à la Twiggy.

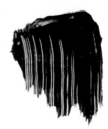

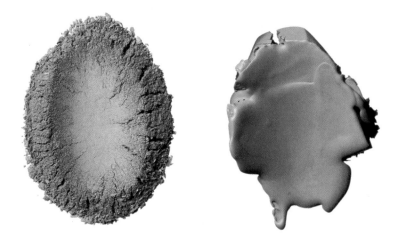

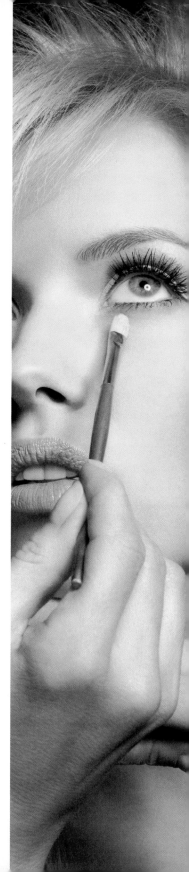

- Now apply a soft nude blush on the apples of the cheeks.

- Finish with nude lipstick; make sure it is a gleamy, slightly shimmering nude. A heavy matte opaque will look dated.

Best Nude Lip Colors for This Look

Fair skin should wear *peachy-pink beiges*.
Medium skin is radiant in *tawny beiges*.
Dark skin will look super sexy with *caramel browns*.

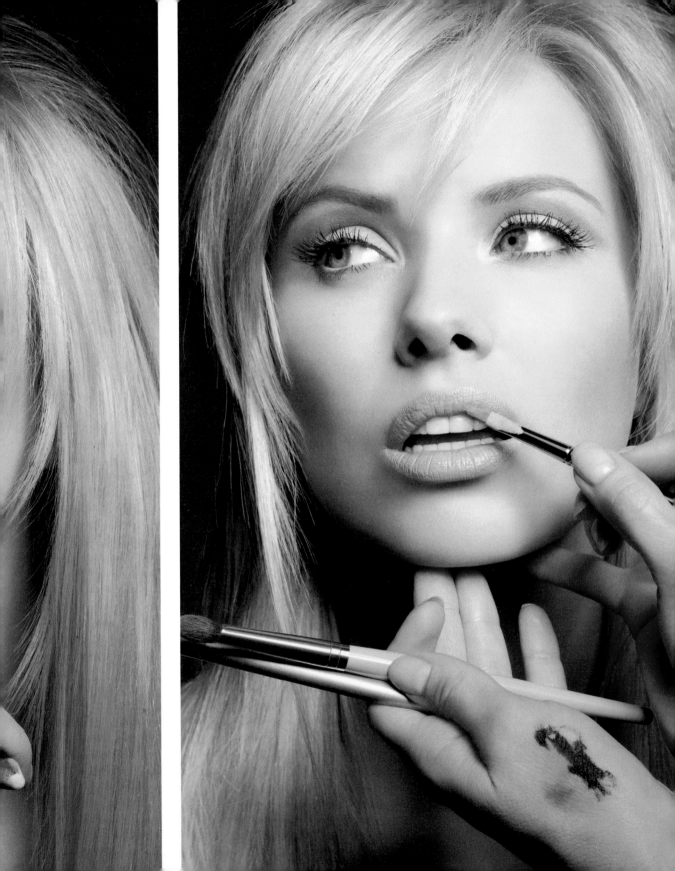

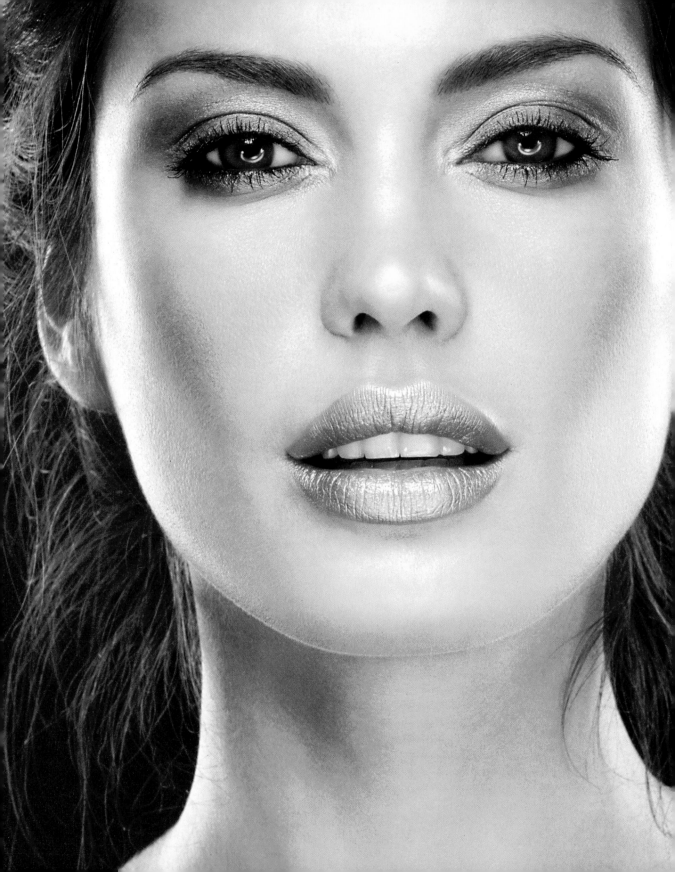

BRONZE GODDESS

The sun-kissed glow is here to stay year-round, and anyone can wear it! To get the best results from a bronzed look, be sure your makeup palette works with your natural coloring. If you have porcelain skin, you won't look natural done up like a Brazilian supermodel. A healthy light glow is a lot more flattering and natural. Likewise, if you're naturally dark, be careful not to end up looking like a gilded bronze statue. Sheer shades are best with this trend, and apply makeup sparingly for a beautiful finish. Details follow.

Get the Look

Begin by mixing in a little gold shimmer to your foundation. Follow the first four steps of the 5-minute face: foundation, under-eye concealer, spot concealer, and powder.

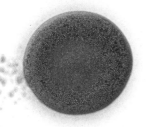

- Now, apply a bronzer to your temples and along your cheekbones.

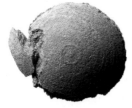

- Dust tawny blush onto the apples of your cheeks.

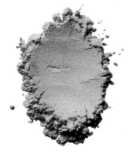

- Dab a little pale gold eye shadow under the arch of each eyebrow and at the inside corner of your eyes.

- Add bronze eye shadow across your lid from lash line to crease.

- Apply black mascara on top and bottom lashes.

- Finish with a slick of sheer bronze lipstick.

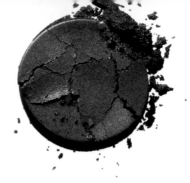

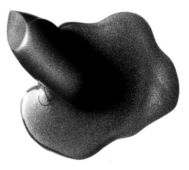

Best Bronzer Shades
Porcelain skin, use a *peachy light bronze.*
Medium skin, think *tawny or terracotta bronze.*
Darker skin tones, choose *deep bronze and copper.*

Best Bronzer Textures
Dry skin, use *creams and sticks.*
Oily to normal skin, use *gels, powders, or aerosols.*

Best Eye Colors to Pair with a Bronzy Look
Blue eyes, try *bronzy gold.*
Brown eyes, try *deep bronze.*
Green eyes, try *burgundy bronze.*
Hazel eyes, try *coppery gold.*

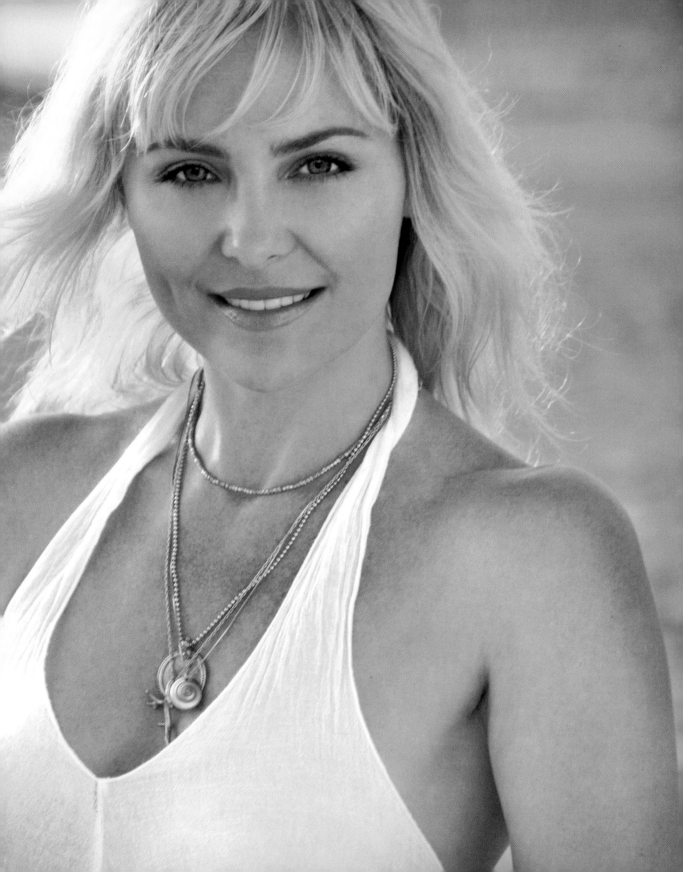

JEWEL TONES

This rich trend usually comes around during the cool fall and winter months, as it allows you to spice up your look and create a little drama. Colors like shimmering jade, amethyst, sapphire, emerald, and turquoise can be worn in many ways, but start simple and work your way up to a more daring style. This is definitely a nighttime look.

Get the Look

Start by applying all nine steps of the 5-minute face: foundation, under-eye concealer, spot concealer, powder, highlighter, blush, eyeliner, mascara, and lip color.

- Sweep a shimmering gem-colored eye shadow under the *lower* lash line.

- Apply a different jewel-toned eye shadow from your lash line to the crease. Start with a sheer wash of color, and build up in layers to reach the intensity you want.

- Last, line the inside rim of your eyes with black pencil. (Have small eyes? Skip this step.)

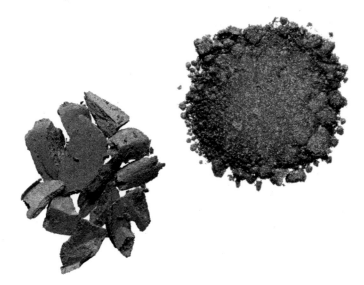

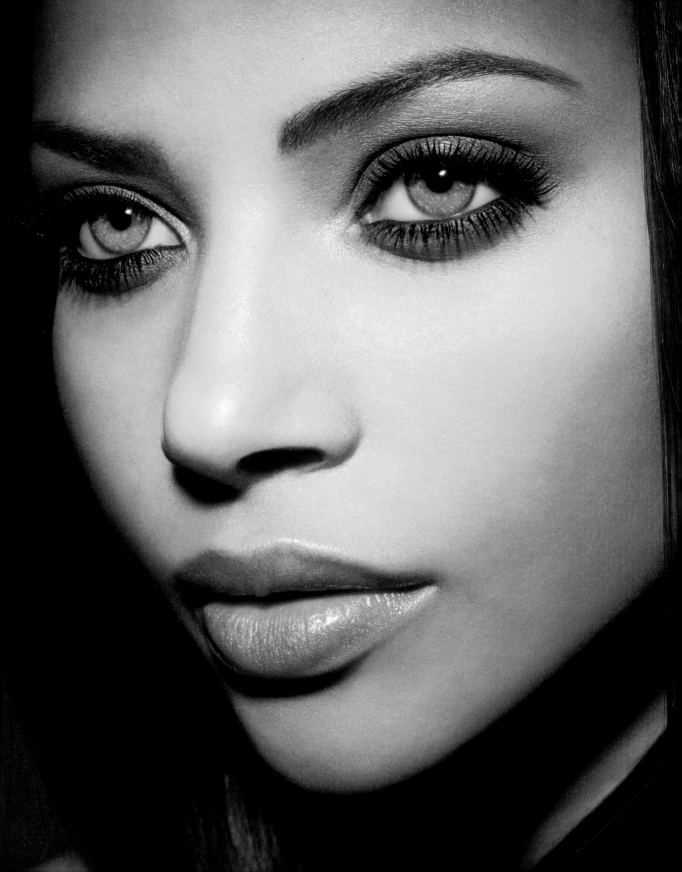

Bold Shadow Tip

You may find that one sheer sweep of this shade will be all you need.

Best Jewel Tones for You

You should feel free to use whatever colors you are drawn to—even choose to wear two at the same time—but if you're not sure, here are some tips for starting out.

Brown eyes totally pop with *sapphire*.
Green eyes are amazing with an *amethyst* shade.
Blue eyes look magical with *jade*.
Hazel eyes look incredible with *jade or emerald*.

METALLICS

Metallic makeup is a trend that lasts because applying it is like putting on a great accessory. A sweep of silver eye shadow or a swipe of golden gloss can make you feel like a goddess. Creams and sheer formulas are easier to wear because they allow your skin to show through, but more intense powders and liners can make a powerful statement when worn on a bare face. When picking metallics, look for refined shimmers rather than glitter to avoid looking like a disco ball. Choose one area to play with the metallics; try highlighting your cheekbones with gold or accentuating your eyes with silver. If you use metallics on eyes, cheeks, *and* lips you run the risk of looking like the Tin Man.

Get the Look

Apply the first nine steps of the 5-minute face: foundation, under-eye concealer, spot concealer, powder, highlighter, blush, eyeliner, mascara, and lip color.

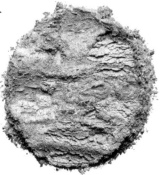

- Next, apply a silver (or whatever metallic color is best for you) eye shadow from your lash line to the crease.

- Apply a small bit of metallic eye shadow under your lower lash line.

- *Voilà!* You're done!

Balancing Act

Remember, apply metallic makeup to *one* area of your face only—keep the rest of your face fairly neutral. When playing with this trend, I like to keep the eyes the focus. Opt for tawny and rosy browns on lips and cheeks. Metallic lips are hard to pull off.

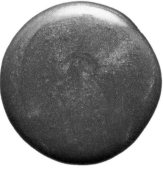

Best Metallic Colors

Light skin tones look super in *silvers and platinum.*

Olive skin tones can totally pull off *bronzes and golds.*

Very dark skin can wear any of these hues!

Fast Fix

For an easy way to experiment with metallic makeup, apply a spot of silver on the center of the upper lid. Or try a speck of gold on the inside corners of your eyes to make them look bright and sparkling. Either will look magical at night and will make your eyes appear bigger.

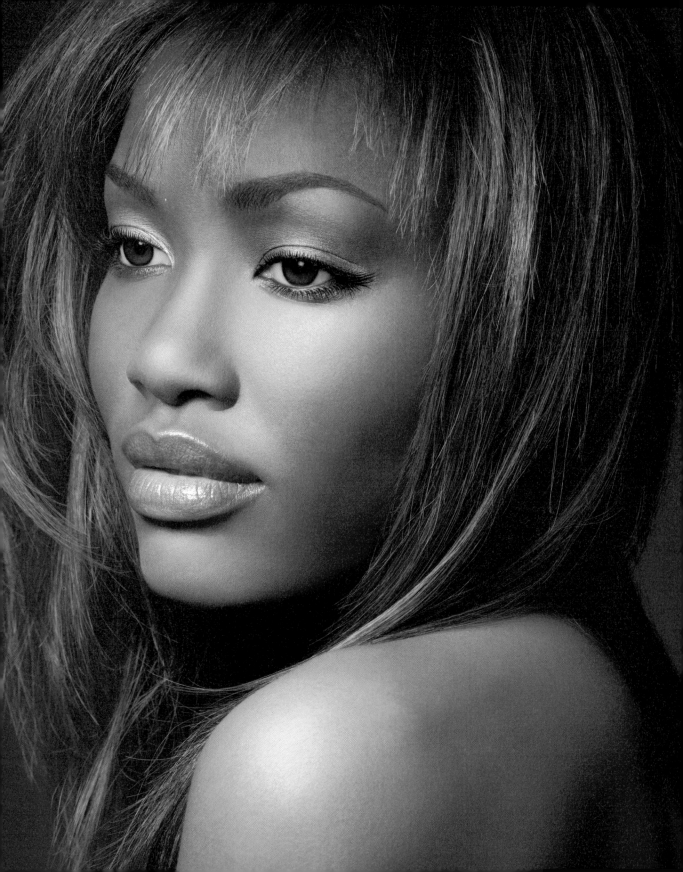

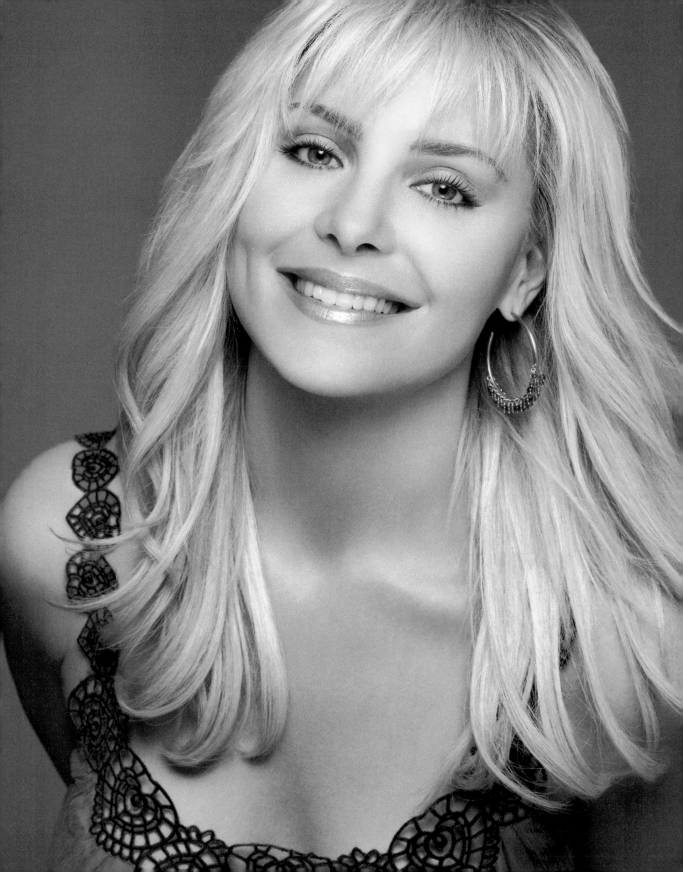

CONGRATULATIONS, LADIES.

You're now armed with all the tools you need to create your most gorgeous 5-minute face.

But let me tell you one last little secret: You were beautiful before you even picked up this book, you are beautiful now as you consider new ways to present yourself to the world, and you will be beautiful every day of your life. Own that beauty that only you possess and you will be the height of loveliness.

Love,
Carmindy

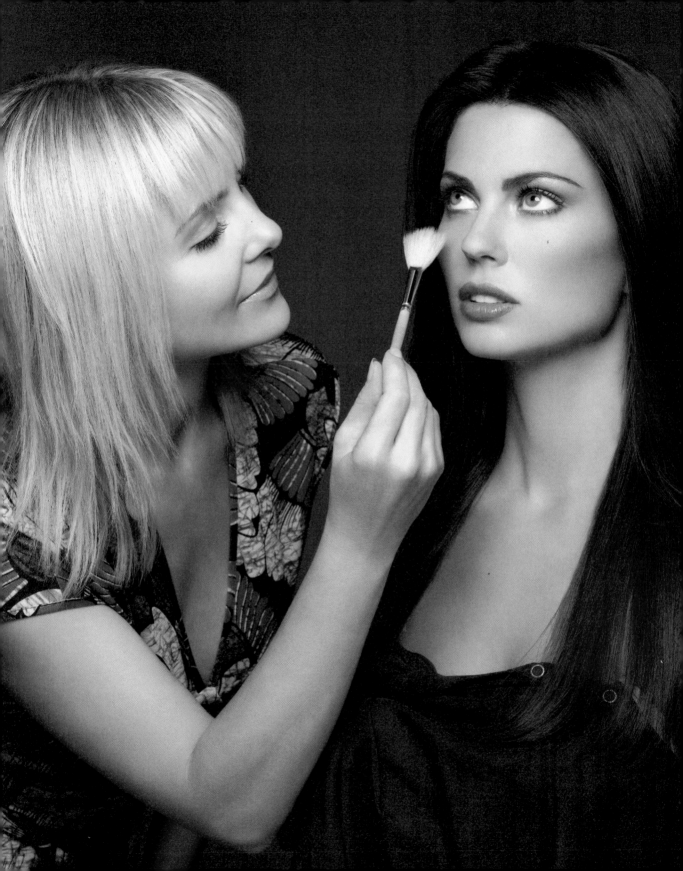

SHOPPING GUIDE

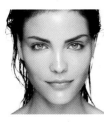

chapter one
SKIN ESSENTIALS

Oily Skin Cleanser

$$$ Estée Lauder Sparkling Clean Oil-Control Foaming Gel Cleanser

$ L'Oréal Paris Ideal Balance Foaming Gel Cleanser

Oily Skin Moisturizer

$$$ NeoStrata Ultra Daytime Skin Smoothing Cream AHA 10 SPF 15

$ Neutrogena Oil-Free Moisturizer

Acne Treatment

$$$ NeoStrata Neoceuticals Acne Spot Treatment Gel

$ Clean and Clear Clear Advantage Acne Spot Treatment

Normal-Combination Skin Cleanser

$$$ Dr. Haushka Cleansing Milk

$ Cetaphil Gentle Skin Cleanser for Normal Skin to Oily Skin

Normal-Combination Skin Moisturizer

$$$ DDF Daily Protective Moisturizer SPF 15

$ Ponds Smooth Perfection Moisturizer

Dry Skin Cleanser

$$$ La Mer The Cleansing Fluid

$ Cetaphil Gentle Skin Cleanser

Dry Skin Moisturizer

$$$ Kiehl's Creme D'Elegance Repairateur

$ Olay Active Hydrating Cream

Eye Makeup Remover

$$$ Longcils Boncza Eye Makeup Remover Pads

$ Almay Moisturizing Eye Makeup Remover Pads

Eye Cream

$$$ La Mer The Eye Balm

$ Neutrogena Healthy Skin Eye Cream

Toners

$$$ Kiehl's Cucumber Herbal Alcohol-Free Toner

$ Burt's Bees Rosewater and Glycerin Toner

Sunscreen

$$$ DDF Organic Sun Protection SPF 30

$ Neutrogena Ultra Sheer Dry Touch Sunblock SPF 30

Exfoliators

$$$ Gly Derm Lotion Lite

$ Alpha Hydrox AHA Enhanced Anti-Wrinkle Exfoliant Cream

Lip Balm

$$$ Kiehl's Lip Balm #1

$ Smith's Rosebud Lip Salve

Self-Tanners

$$$ Pout Sexy Sunwear Ultimate Fake Tan

$ Jergens Natural Glow Daily Moisturizer

Body Lotion/Shimmer

$$$ Stila All Over Shimmer Liquid Luminizer

$ Neutrogena Shimmer Sheers

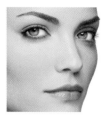

chapter two

GET BROWS THAT WOW

Tweezers

$$$ Tweezerman Tweezers

$ LaCross Exacta Tweeze Tweezers

Manicure Scissors

$$$ Tweezerman Scissors

$ Mira Cuticle Scissors

Brow Brush

$$$ Stila # 18 Double-Sided Brow Brush

$ e.l.f. Professional Eyelash and Brow Wand

Brow Pencil

$$$ Givenchy Eyebrow Show Powdery Eyebrow Pencil

$ Avon Glimmersticks Brow Definer

Brow Powder

$$$ Anastasia Brow Powder Duo

$ Ardell Brow Defining Powder

Brow Groomer

$$$ Dior Gel Fixateur Brow Gel

$ Revlon Brow Fantasy Pencil and Gel

Waterproof Liquid Brow Color

$$$ Makeup Forever Brow Corrector

$ Corey Cosmetics Eye Fix-Sation Brow Wax

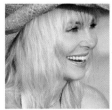

chapter three

FOUNDATION, CONCEALER, AND POWDER

Tinted Moisturizer

$$$ Laura Mercier Tinted Moisturizer

$ Neutrogena Healthy Skin Enhancer

Liquid Foundation

$$$ Makeup Forever Face and Body Liquid Makeup

$ L'Oréal Paris True Match Super-Blendable Makeup

Cream Foundation

$$$ Cinema Secrets Ultimate Foundation

$ Avon Beyond Color Skin Smoothing Foundation

Mineral Powder Foundation

$$$ Bare Escentuals i.d. BareMinerals Foundation

$ L'Oréal Paris Bare Naturale Powder Mineral Foundation

Aerosol Spray Foundation

$$$ Era Face Spray On Foundation by Classified Cosmetics

$ Sally Hansen Airbrush Makeup Spray

Sponges

$ Posh by Upstage Non-Latex Makeup Wedges

Primer

$$$ Era Primer by Classified Cosmetics

$ Sephora Professional Perfection Makeup Base

Mattifyer

$$$ OC Eight Mattifying Gel

$ The Body Shop Tea Tree Oil Mattifying Moisture Gel

Under-Eye Concealer

$$$ Benefit Eye Bright

$ The Body Shop Concealer Pencil

Concealer for Blemishes, Scars, Veins, and Sunspots

$$$ Stila Cover Up Stick

$ Revlon Color Stay Blemish Concealer

Powder

$$$ M.A.C. Blot Powder

$ Cover Girl Clean Fragrance-Free Pressed Powder

Blotting Papers

$$$ Lancôme Matte Finish Shine Control Blotting Sheets

$ Clean And Clear Oil Absorbing Sheets

chapter five

THE BEST MAKEUP COLORS FOR YOUR SKIN TONE

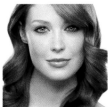 **PORCELAIN-SKINNED REDHEAD**

Highlighter

$$$ Bare Escentuals Glimmers in "2000"

$ La Femme Sparkle Dust in "21"

Eyeliner

$$$ Sue Devitt Eye Intensifier Pencil in "Tanzania"

$ Almay Intense I-Color Eyeliner in "Brown Topaz"

Blush

$$$ M.A.C. Blushcream in "Lilicent"

$ Revlon Cream Blush in "Just Peachy"

Lip Gloss

$$$ Jouer Lip Gloss in "Ginger"

$ L'Oréal Paris Colour Juice in "Iced Latte"

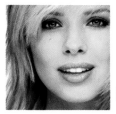

BLONDE

Highlight

$$$ Makeup Forever Diamond Cream in "2"

$ Jane Glimmeratzi Eye Gloss in "Diamond-Eyezed"

Eyeliner

$$$ Benefit Eye Sketching Pencil in "Royale"

$ Almay Intense i-Color in "Amethyst"

Eye Shadow

$$$ M.A.C. Eye Shadow in "Shale"

$ Neutrogena Mineral Sheers in "Clay"

Blush

$$$ Body and Soul Rouge in Madagascar Pink

$ Revlon Powder Blush in "Love That Pink"

Lip Gloss

$$$ Bourjois Effect 3D Lipgloss in "5"

$ Styli-Style Plastique High Shine Lipgloss in "Wild Martini"

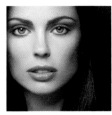

BRUNETTE

Highlighter
$$$ Lancôme Color Design Eye Shadow in "Gaze"

$ Maybelline Shadow Stylist Eye Shadow in "Elegant Pearl"

Eye Shadow
$$$ M.A.C. Eye Shadow in "Satin Taupe"

$ e.l.f. Custom Eyes in "Dusk"

Eye Shadow
$$$ Laura Mercier Eye Colour in "Truffle"

$ Maybelline Expert Wear Eye Shadow in "Crème De Cocoa"

Blush
$$$ Lorac Blush in "Plum"

$ N.Y.C. Powder Blush in "Outside Café"

Lipstick
$$$ Lorac Cream Lipstick in "Wild Orchid"

$ Milani Lipstick in "Rose Fetish"

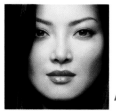

ASIAN

Lash Curler

$$$ Japonesque Precision Lash Curler

$ Tweezerman Professional Corner Lash Curler

Highlight

$$$ Bobbi Brown Shimmer Brick in "Pink"

$ L'Oréal Paris Illumination Loose Eye Color in "Dawn"

Eye Shadow

$$$ Smashbox Eyeshadow in "Flatscreen"

$ Maybelline Expert Wear Eye Shadow Duo in "Indian Summer"

Eyeliner

$$$ Chanel Aqua Crayon Eye Colour Stick in "Very Black"

$ Almay Eyeliner in "Black"

Cream Color

$$$ Paula Dorf Cheek Color Cream in "Candy Apple"

$ Revlon Cream Blush in "Blushing Mauve"

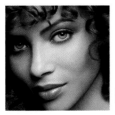

MOCHA SKIN

Highlight
$$$ Nars Duo Eyeshadow in "Bohemian Gold"

$ N.Y.C. Sparkle Dust Eyeshadow in "893"

Eye Shadow
$$$ M.A.C. Eye Shadow in "Woodwinked"

$ Milani Eyeshadow in "Golden Bronze"

Eye Shadow
$$$ Body and Soul Eyeshadow in "Volcano"

$ NYX Single Eyeshadow in "Walnut Bronze"

Blush
$$$ Benefit Dallas Powder

$ Milani Powder Bronzer in "2"

Lip Gloss
$$$ Lancôme Fever Gloss in "Heatstroke"

$ Milani Glitz Glamour Gloss in "Lady Like"

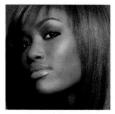

DARK SKIN

Highlight

$$$ Nars Cream Blush in "Gold Member"

$ L'Oréal Paris Crystal Infinite Sparkling Eye Shadow Cream in "Champagne"

Eyeliner

$$$ Dior Crayon Eyeliner Waterproof in "Captivating Blue"

$ Styli-Style Eyeliner in "Navy/Marine"

Blush

$$$ M.A.C. Blush in "Loverush"

$ Black Radiance Blush in "Spiced Ginger"

Lip Gloss

$$$ Dior Addict Ultra Gloss Reflect in "A Stitch of Brown #627"

$ Milani Lipgloss in "Baby Doll"

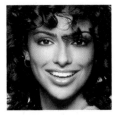

OLIVE SKIN

Highlight

$$$ Face Stockholm Eye Dust in "Vanity"

$ La Femme Sparkle Dust in "9"

Eye Shadow

$$$ M.A.C. Pigment Color Powder in "Chocolate Brown"

$ Maybelline Shadow Stylist Eye Shadow in "Sleek Brown"

Blush

$$$ M.A.C. Blush in "Fleur Power"

$ Cover Girl Classic Blush in "Rose Silk"

Lip Gloss

$$$ Lorac Lotsa Lip in "Babie"

$ Milani Glitzy Glamour Gloss in "Glitz + Glam"

chapter six

BEAUTIFUL AT EVERY AGE

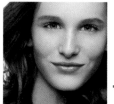 **TEENS**

Eye Shadow

$$$ Pop Beauty Eye Cakes in "Bright Blue"

$ Maybelline Shadow Stylist Eye Shadow in "Trendy Blue"

Colored Mascara

$$$ Cargo SuperEyes Mascara

$ Almay Intense i-Color Bring Out Lengthening Mascara

Blush

$$$ Pout Blush in "Berry Babe"

$ NYX Blush in "Pinky"

Lip Gloss

$$$ Sue Devitt Lip Gloss in "Nantucket"

$ Jane Lip Sauce in "Strawberry Cream"

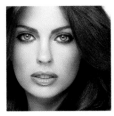

TWENTIES

Eye Shadow

$$$ M.A.C. Eye Shadow in "Vex"

$ Neutrogena Mineral Sheers in "Stone"

Liquid Eyeliner

$$$ Makeup Forever Color Liner in "26"

$ Prestige Liquid Eyeliner in "Icon"

Lip Gloss

$$$ Cargo Lip Gloss Duo in "Bonbon"

$ N.Y.C. Liquid Lip Shine in "Cherrywood"

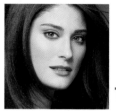

THIRTIES

Eyeliner/Powder

$$$ Cargo Smoky Eye Eyeliner Duo in "Barcelona"

$ L'Oréal Paris HIP Pure Pigment Shadow Stick in "Mesmerizing"

Blush

$$$ Nars Blush in "Outlaw"

$ Avon True Color Blush in "Rose Lustre"

Lip Gloss

$$$ Jouer Lip Gloss in "Breeze"

$ Cover Girl WetSlicks in "Wine Shine"

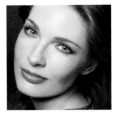

FORTIES

Luminizers
$$$ Benefit Highbeam

$ Wild and Wild MegaGlow Face Illuminator in "Blushing"

Eye Shadow
$$$ Laura Mercier Eye Colour in "Vanilla Nuts"

$ Cover Girl Eye Enhancers in "French Vanilla"

Eye Shadow
$$$ M.A.C. Eye Shadow in "Haux"

$ L'Oréal Paris Wear Infinite Eyeshadow in "503"

Eyeliner
$$$ Chanel Stylo Yeux Waterproof Long Lasting Eyeliner in "Espresso"

$ Physicians Formula Eye Definer Automatic Eye Pencil in "Dark Brown"

Blush
$$$ Cargo Blush in "The Big Easy"

$ Jane Blushing Cheeks in "Blushing Earth"

Lipstick
$$$ M.A.C. Lipstick in "Viva Glam V"

$ Cover Girl Continuous Color Lipstick in "Sugar Almond"

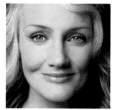

FIFTIES

Eye Shadow
$$$ Lancôme Colour Design Eyeshadow in "Click"

$ Cover Girl Eye Enhancers in "Tapestry Taupe"

Eyeliner
$$$ Dior Crayon Liner Waterproof in "Intense Brown"

$ Avon Ultra Luxury Eyeliner in "Dark Brown"

Blush
$$$ Stila Blush in "Rose"

$ Cover Girl Cheekers in "Natural Twinkle"

Lip Liner
$$$ Guerlain Divinora Lip Pencil in "42 Beige Nuetre"

$ Cover Grl Outlast Smoothwear Lip Liner in Nude

Lipstick
$$$ Guerlain Kiss Kiss Lipstick in "544 Reve d'Or"

$ L'Oréal Paris Colour Riche Lipstick in "Tender Pink"

Waterproof Mascara
$$$ Shu Uemura Precise Volume Mascara Waterproof

$ Maybelline Lash Discovery Waterproof

The 5-Second Face-lift
$$$ Benefit Eye Bright

$ The Body Shop Concealer Pencil

chapter seven
SPECIAL OCCASION LOOKS

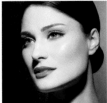 ## CLASSIC BLACK-TIE PARTY

False Lashes

$$$ Shu Uemura False Eyelashes in "01"

$ Andrea ModLash in "53"

Cream Eyeliner

$$$ Smashbox Cream Eyeliner in "Caviar"

$ Paula's Choice Constant Color Gel Eyeliner in "Nightfall"

Lipstick

$$$ Givenchy Rouge Interdit Lipstick in "18 Elegant Rouge"

$ Revlon Super Lustrous Lipstick in "Love That Red"

Lipstain

$$$ Benefit Benetint

$ Styli-Style L3 Lip Stain

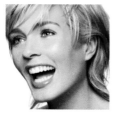

VACATION GLOW

Bronzer
$$$ Youngblood Mineral Radiance in "Sundance"

$ Neutrogena Shimmer Sheers in "Mystified"

Eye Shadow
$$$ Bare Escentuals Glimmers in "True Gold"

$ La Femme Sparkle Dust in "1"

Blush
$$$ Lorac Blush in "Desire"

$ L'Oréal Paris Blush Délice in "Strawberry Tart"

Lip Gloss
$$$ M.A.C. Lustreglass Lip Gloss in "Budding"

$ Styli-Style Plastique High Shine Lip Gloss in "Mambo"

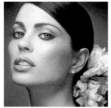

WEDDING

Eye Shadow

$$$ M.A.C. Eye Shadow in "Velum"

$ N.Y.C. Iridescent Sparkle Eye Dust in "891 Opal Sparkle"

Eyeliner

$$$ Sue Devitt Eye Intensifier Pencil in "Zaire"

$ Revlon Color Stay Eye Liner in "Vixen"

Blush

$$$ Bourjois Blush in "Rose D'or"

$ Maybelline Expert Wear Blush in "Gentle Rose"

Lip Gloss

$$$ Nars Lip Lacquer in "Baby Doll"

$ Jordana InColor Lip Jelly Juice Tints in "Strawberries and Cream"

Body Glow

$$$ Body and Soul Glitz Moisturizer

$ Nivea Body Silky Shimmer Lotion

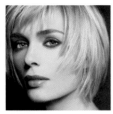

TAKE YOUR LOOK FROM DAY TO NIGHT

Eyeliner

$$$ Sue Devitt Eye Intensifier Pencil in "Pointe Noir"

$ Prestige Soft Blend Kohl Eye Liner in "Jet Black"

Eye Shadow

$$$ Stila Eye Shadow Pan Shadows in "Barefoot Contessa"

$ L'Oréal Paris Wear Infinite Eye Shadow in "Satin Taupe"

Lipstick

$$$ M.A.C. Frost Lipstick in "Plastique"

$ N.Y.C. Ultra Last Lipwear in "Brandy Sparkle"

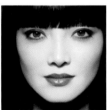

HOLIDAY FACE

Eye Shadow

$$$ Laura Mercier Eye Colour Shimmer in "Chambord"

$ Cover Girl Eye Enhancers Eyeshadow in "Forever Fig"

Lipstick

$$$ Nars Lipstick in "Scarlet Empress"

$ L'Oréal Paris HIP Lipstick in "Merry"

chapter eight

TRENDS THAT WORK

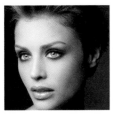

SMOKY EYES

Dark Eye Shadow

$$$ Nars Eye Shadow in "Night Breed"

$ Milani Eye Shadow in "Storm"

Soft Eye Shadow

$$$ M.A.C. Eye Shadow in "Beauty Marked"

$ Jordana Eye Shadow Pot in "Wine"

Lip Gloss

$$$ Dior Addict Ultra-Gloss in "483"

$ Styli-Style Plastique High Shine Lipgloss in "Sexy Martini"

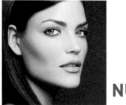

NUDES

Eye Shadow Compact

$$$ Dior 5 Color Eye Shadow in "Incognito"

$ Maybelline Expert Wear Shadow Quads in "Designer Chocolates"

Blush

$$$ Shu Uemura Glow On Blush in "M Amber 89"

$ APT 5 Blush in "B-1"

Lipstick

$$$ Lancôme Color Design Lipstick in "Natural Beauty"

$ Revlon Super Lustrous Lipstick in "Almost Nude"

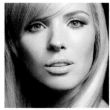

RETRO SIXTIES

Vanilla Eye Shadow

$$$ Makeup Forever Eye Shadow in "000"

$ Jane Eye Zing in "White Lies"

Taupe Eye Shadow

$$$ Body and Soul Eye Shadow in "Sultry"

$ Maybelline Expert Wear Eye Shadow in "Utaupia"

Mascara

$$$ Dior DiorShow Mascara in "Black"

$ Maybelline Great Lash in "Blackest Black"

Blush

$$$ Bobbi Brown Blush in "Spice"

$ N.Y.C. Powder Blush in "Sutton Place"

Lipstick

$$$ Body and Soul Lipstick in "Dew"

$ Neutrogena Lip Boost Lipstick in "Sheer Suede"

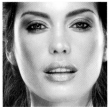

BRONZE GODDESS

Bronzer
$$$ Era Rayz Spray On Bronzer in "3 By The Sea"

$ Physicians Formula Shimmer Strips in "Bronzer"

Gold Eye Shadow
$$$ Face Stockholm Eye Dust in "Vanity"

$ La Femme Sparkle Dust in "9"

Bronze Eye Shadow
$$$ Makeup Forever Star Powder in "930"

$ La Femme Sparkle Dust in "27"

Eyeliner
$$$ M.A.C. Eye Kohl in "Teddy"

$ Prestige Soft Blend Kohl Eyeliner in "Spiced"

Blush
$$$ Guerlain Terracotta Blush & Sun Sheer Bronzing Blush in "03 Suntan"

$ Wet and Wild Bronzzer Compact in "741B Bally Bronze"

Lipstick
$$$ M.A.C. Frost Lipstick in "Bronze Shimmer"

$ Milani High Shine Lip Stick Pencil In "Topaz"

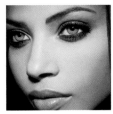

JEWEL TONES

Purple Eye Shadow

$$$ M.A.C. Pigment Color Powder in "Violet"

$ L'Oréal Paris HIP Pure Pigment Shadow Stick in "Violet"

Blue Eye Shadow

$$$ M.A.C. Eye Shadow in "Freshwater"

$ Cover Girl Eye Enhancers in "Aqua Paradise"

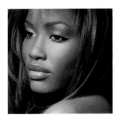

METALLICS

Eye Shadow

$$$ Makeup Forever Star Powder in "948"

$ L'Oréal Paris HIP Pure Pigment Shadow Stick in "Dazzling"

Lip Gloss

$$$ Armani Lip Gloss in "2"

$ Neutrogena Moistureshine Gloss in "25"

ACKNOWLEDGMENTS

The following people made this book possible, and I love and appreciate them more than words can say, but I will try.

Lauren Keller Galit, my agent, who got it from the get-go and hustled it all the way, pregnant and all. You are amazing!

Maureen O'Neal at HarperCollins for having the ultimate faith in me and seeing the vision.

Palma Kolansky, meeting you was one of the biggest gifts in my life. This book was our dream, and we realized it together. The beauty you see in women is powerful. You are an inspiration.

Patrick Melville, Hair God! You are a true artist, and your hard work and dedication to this book was just incredible.

Debbie Shapiro, who is the greatest producer in the world. You worked tirelessly on this project, and I will love you forever for it.

Devon Jarvis, for your willingness to dedicate yourself 100 percent and create such stunning shots.

Mary Rose Almasi, your talent is limitless, thank you for helping me create something we can be proud of.

Valerie Oula, casting agent extraordinaire who always delivered!

Erica Cruz, for all your patience and devotion. "You're fired!" (Just kidding!)

Christine Vono, for all your hair help.

Steven Brown, Francis Catania, Arun Kuplas, and James Gingold, "The boys!" You worked so hard, sometimes double-shifting. You were the framework of this book.

Thank you to my supportive family at **Sun Studios,** our digital artist **Tonino Fodale** (the best in the biz), **Giuseppe Luccardi, Jean Bourbon, Merve Ozal, Dan Wetuk, Evelyn Basa, Darbin Navarro,** and **Daniele Borgia.** You were my cheerleaders and supported us throughout this whole experience.

Allison Berlin, my amazing stylist who saved the day.

Dr. Rosemarie Ingleton, the most gorgeous dermatologist, who has taught me so much about skin and beauty.

Joy Bergman, the lovely wordsmith, for giving me gold.

A huge thank you to the lovely models: **Marie-Claude Guy, Alise Shoemaker, Gabriela Salvado, Jeanette Hallen, Alexandra Fomon, Cinthia Moura, Cindy Joseph, Fabiana Tambosi, Jane Kim, Sophie Meister, Lucy Kemp, Hannah Wane, Kindra Hanson, Denise Vasi, Luciana Curtis,** and **Cassia Regina DeLara.**

I want to thank the designers of **Me&Ro Jewelry, Manon Von Gurkan Jewelry,** and **Nieves Lavi Apparel** for making me feel so beautiful.

A big kiss to my best friend & husband, **Javier Acosta,** who loved and supported me throughout this great experience. Te Amo.

MEET THE TEAM

CARMINDY: MAKEUP

Millions of viewers every week count on Carmindy to teach them the latest makeup tips and tricks on TLC's hit show "What Not to Wear."

Since her Southern California childhood, Carmindy has dreamed of traveling the world doing makeup and meeting inspiring people. Through hard work and an unstoppable attitude, she's made that dream a reality. She's painted faces in the studios of Paris, along the beaches of Brazil, and on the streets of Havana. She's lived in Los Angeles, Milan, Miami, and now makes her home with her husband, Javier, in New York, where she has established herself as a top fashion makeup artist.

Carmindy's work can be seen on the editorial pages of leading magazines such as *Cosmopolitan, Elle, InStyle, O, Essence, Self, Lucky, Seventeen, Marie Claire,* and *Glamour.* Her commercial-campaign clients include Maybelline, Sephora, Clairol, Avon, Aveeno, CoverGirl, Almay, Bath and Body Works, Crest Whitestrips, and Q-tips.

Carmindy is always looking for the next great way to communicate with her fans. She writes a monthly beauty e-newsletter featuring answers to questions submitted through her website www.carmindy.com, and is a freelance beauty writer for several other high-traffic beauty websites.

PALMA KOLANSKY: PHOTOGRAPHER

Palma Kolansky is one of the top fashion and beauty photographers in NYC. In a career that spans over thirty years, working with commercial clients such as Revlon, Clairol, L'Oreal, Maybelline, and Avon, Kolansky has traveled the world shooting top models and celebrities for fashion magazines, album covers, and advertising campaigns. A fine art photographer as well, her collections are shown in galleries, auctioned for charities, and appear in many art publications. She taught photography at the School of Visual Arts and has been a guest lecturer at the Rhode Island School of Design. Recently, she was featured at Princeton University in a presentation called *"The Artist as a Working Man."* Kolansky lives on the East End of Long Island with her husband and teenage son.

PATRICK MELVILLE: HAIR

Patrick Melville has long been considered among the most prestigious hairstylists in the fashion industry. Over the past twenty years he has worked with such magazines as *Vogue, W, Elle,* and *Harper's Bazaar.* He is the creative director of The Patrick Melville Salon at Rockefeller Plaza in NYC, and his clientele includes such high-profile celebrities as Ashley Judd, Catherine Zeta-Jones, Halle Berry, Heidi Klum, Demi Moore, Sharon Stone, Rosario Dawson, Brooke Shields, Sting, Tom Cruise, and Harry Connick Jr. His technical knowledge is unsurpassed, and his ability to collaborate and create wonderful hair with the best artistic teams in fashion and beauty has made him an invaluable asset to the industry. Melville lives in upstate New York with his wife and daughter.

DEVON JARVIS: STILL-LIFE PHOTOGRAPHY

Devon Jarvis is a graduate of the Parsons School of Design in NYC and began his career shooting architectural and interior photography on locations around the world. His still-life photography clients include *Self, O, InStyle, Parents, Fitness, Women's Health,* and *Cookie* magazines. His creative eye and impeccable skills in capturing texture, form, and color make him one of the most sought-after in the field. Jarvis lives in Brooklyn, New York, with his wife and two children.

OPPOSITE PAGE: PATRICK MELVILLE, CARMINDY, AND PALMA KOLANSKY

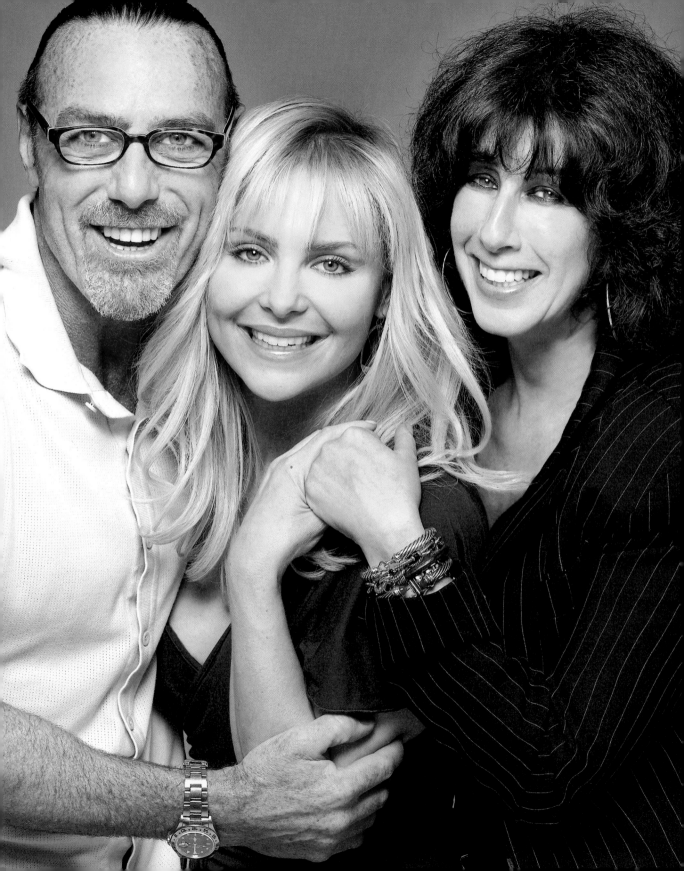